In Love Forever™

In Love Forever™

7 Secrets to a Joyous, Juicy Relationship

Cary & Wendy Valentine

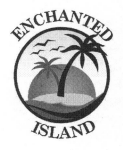

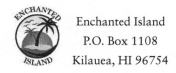

Enchanted Island
P.O. Box 1108
Kilauea, HI 96754

WeCare@InLoveForever.com
www.CaryValentine.net

Cover design: Paul Bond (www.PaulBondArt.com)
Interior design: Adan Garcia & Lee Binder
Edited: Finesse Writing and Editing LLC & Jeri Lynne Stewart
Romantic Day (Tropic Version) Painting: Jim Warren
Lotus Flower: Bahman Farzad

Library of Congress Cataloging-in-Publication Data:
2014949850

ISBN 978-0692279304

ISBN 069227930X

Printed in the United States of America

"We are weaned from our timidity
In the flush of love's light
we dare be brave
And suddenly we see
that love costs all we are
and will ever be.
Yet it is only love
which sets us free."

– Maya Angelou

A joyous, juicy relationship
occurs by choice, not by chance.

Secrets of love are hidden within you,
waiting to be discovered
when you go looking for them.

We thank our parents, extended family, siblings, and their families – Jane, Julie, Chuck, Stu, Neil, and Larry – for their love and support.

A heartfelt thank you to Heather and Dan Jordan for the arduous journey teaching us about the power of choice. Without you both, this book would have never been realized.

Grandma Mary, thank you for being Cary's angel.

We want to thank our dear friends from all over the globe, too many to name here, yet you know who you are.

We are very grateful for the exceptional abilities of our editorial and artistic team: Lee Binder, Paul Bond, Adan Garcia, Julia Hall, Jeri Lynne Stewart, Tracy Ann Teel, and Bobby Vilas.

The highest gratitude for The Creator, God, that has produced everything on beautiful Earth and given us all the chance to transform our misery into living passionate, heartfelt lives.

We also want to thank a select group (since this list can go on for pages) that have influenced our lives: Julie Andrews, St. Francis & St. Claire of Assisi, Frank Baum, Lenny Blank, Andrea Bocelli, Gautama Buddha, Leo Buscaglia, Jim Carrey, Kripalu Center, Deepak Chopra, Stewart Cink, Kevin Costner, Salvador Dali, Leonardo DiCaprio, Celine Dion, Amrit Desai, Danny Devito, Walt Disney, David Feherty, Albert Finney, Morgan Freeman, Mahatma Gandhi, Marvin Gaye, Khalil Gibran, S.N. Goenka & Vipassana Mediation, Alex Haley, Skip Hadden, Tom Hanks, Whitney Houston, Ron Howard, Martin Luther King, Jr, Coretta Scott King, Gypsy Kings, Kripalvananda (Bapuji), Peter Jackson, Jesus, Dr. Vasant Lad, George Lucas, Makana, Nelson Mandela, Tug McGraw, Airto Moreira, Moses, Rafael Nadal, Milton Nascimento, Babatunde Olatunji, Tony Osanah, Maxfield Parrish, John Ramsay, Keali'i Reichel, Rumi, Rush, Susan Sarandon, Sir Ernest Shackleton, Florence Scovel Shinn, Will Smith, Sylvester Stallone, Cat Stevens, Patrick Stewart, Noel Paul Stookey & family, Henry Augustine Tate, Shirley Temple, J.R.R. Tolkien, John Travolta, Robin Williams, Marianne Williamson, Oprah Winfrey, Caetano Veloso, Barry White, Tiger Woods, Franco Zeffirelli.

Mahalo nui loa to the enchanting island of Kaua'i and our Ohana.

Table of Contents

Chapter 7

Chapter 8

Chapter 9

Prologue

After spending a few hours on the lanai enjoying watching the humpback whales breach out of the water all afternoon, Wendy came inside, in her wheelchair, as she was no longer able to lift her body.

During the afternoon, Wendy seemed to come to terms with her life, which had been a constant battle the last two years, and she calmly and suddenly announced to me that she was going to pass on soon. Her body suddenly went weak. Looking at Dave, her nurse, I wondered if she was going to pass right then. She survived that night, yet, in the two subsequent weekends, we found ourselves in the ambulance headed to the emergency room at Wilcox Hospital.

That second weekend in the hospital, Wendy stopped speaking completely. After many tests, it was determined that Wendy should go home. Her two-year battle with glioblastoma multiforme, the most aggressive type of brain tumor, was soon coming to an end. When I was told by the doctors there was nothing more to be done, the weight of this two year pursuit came crashing down on me. All the trips to the hospitals, all the fights with the insurance company for Wendy to receive alternative and groundbreaking treatments from the Burzynski Clinic in Houston and UCSD, which kept her alive with a quality of life far longer than her initial physicians told her she would live.

I called my brother, Neil, a chiropractor, and his wife, Sabine, a neonatal nurse, who both offered us tremendous support during this ordeal. In an explosion of emotions, I said, "What the f*** was this all for? Spending so much time, money, and resources to still have her die?"

I was overcome by the intense realization that throughout this two-year period I had believed that Wendy would be able to overcome this tremendous disease ... and she was now suddenly being taken from me. Wendy's brain surgeon told me that we were given at least an extra year, more than what he would have ever believed was possible.

I was amazed how Wendy always kept a positive attitude after going through many trials, tribulations, and challenges with this brain tumor. In the two years that I was constantly by her side as her caregiver, I frequently watched her nurses leave the room in tears due to how much joyous love Wendy offered them.

But the time had come, as Wendy predicted, and in the middle of the night on March 11th, two years and one day to her diagnosis, Wendy peacefully passed on. I was amazed at how quickly the life force left her body, and how her skin lost its color.

I, and a very caring hospice nurse, bathed her, placed a tiara on her precious head, and dressed her in a princess dress before her body was taken to the crematorium. Wendy was a princess of love; she offered so much to both children and adults as a life long international teacher. Her angelic voice accompanied by her acoustic guitar and ukulele were often heard in elementary schools, art classes, and on stages throughout Brazil and the U.S.

My life has been forever enhanced by the 24 years in which we loved, fell out of love, stood at the brink of divorce, and crawled and begged our way back to more juicy love than either one of us had ever experienced before.

The first version of this book that we wrote together was completed just weeks before her initial diagnosis. Our story is the end result of our journey of blood, sweat, and tears that took us from Massachusetts, Brazil, New Mexico, Colorado, Idaho, Vermont, and finally Hawaii. An adventure that revealed the keys to truly being *In Love Forever.* These are the keys that helped pull me out of the deep grief I experienced when Wendy passed. As I was rebooting my life, I asked myself, "What do I want to do now?" And after I explored many options, it became very clear to me that my strongest desire and joy was to assist people with letting go of their pain, so they could have better relationships as couples and be more accepting and joyous as individuals. Every moment is precious, and I am very excited that you are about to read and take an irresistible, juicy journey with us to explore new states of joyous love for yourself and your partner.

Aloha 'oe, Wendy. Two years exactly to your passing, this book serves as a living legacy to the beautiful life you led and is now touching and transforming multitudes of folks around the globe; your impact and courage to lead a life way off the beaten path and to discover the secrets to true happiness continue to help others. Wendy, I cherish you as your mate and fellow traveler. Thank you for your encouragement to continue on and offer this to others.

I am now bestowed with the honor of sharing this book with you who are reading this as a guide. You don't have to experience the many difficult years it took us to figure out and realize "how-to" have a lasting, juicy relationship. This book will quickly transform the pain or discomfort you're experiencing into truly having the relationship and life of your dreams.

Cary Valentine
March 11, 2014

About Us – A True Story of Transformation

In our 24 years together, Wendy and I went from a paradise where we were giddy in love to a hellish, dark place on the brink of divorce. Miraculously, we found our way out of a relationship nightmare and became more in love than ever before. Here's our real story of transformation.

In 2001, I was depressed, worried about money, losing weight, unsure of my future, not making love with my wife, and living a silent hell. I felt dissatisfied and disconnected in my own home, but to the outside world, I acted as though everything was "just fine." Wendy and I were not able to be honest about our feelings. I woke up one morning, looked at Wendy, and thought, "Who are you?" I felt empty. I felt no connection to her. I went to play basketball that day, alone. I thought to myself, "What do I have to lose if I'm not with her?" I was afraid to be alone, but suddenly I recognized I was already alone.

My unhappiness came as a shock to Wendy. She was consumed with doubts about her looks and was keeping it shockingly secret.

Unknowingly, we had been dampening our zest for life, for each other, and our talents. We were not working well as an intimate team and were not flourishing financially. And we certainly were not juicy! We didn't realize how unhappy we were and how many secrets we had been keeping from ourselves and each other until we hit rock bottom. Our lives clearly were not working.

Searching for answers to get out of our misery, we hit a wall. We had already tried a variety of therapies to erase the pain: yoga, silent meditation retreats, fasting, organic diets, couples counseling, and therapy. At the time, we owned and managed a health spa in the Rocky Mountains of Colorado, where we gave enough enemas to last a lifetime! Although each therapy and circumstance was helpful in its own way, we were humbled by a continuous deep feeling of unhappiness.

We had reached a point where we were physically and emotionally sick of our judgmental, unhappy patterns. This is when our lives began to shift. Help came in a serendipitous way. Two dear, old friends called and invited us to simplify our lives by working with them on their 80-acre wildlife refuge. This led us *on a four year quest in the Idaho desert, where our only other acquaintances, besides our two friends, were rattlesnakes, coyotes, badgers, deer ... and our own two cats! Initially (needless to say), we were frightened by the rattlesnakes and the coyotes, but believe it or not, we learned to befriend them!*

During our very intense work in Idaho, I remember so well the day that I came to Wendy in tears expressing how I longed for just 24 hours without this thick, black cloud of despair and constant battling of doubts hovering over me. I was like "Pig-Pen" in the Peanuts cartoon, who was often depicted with a cloud of dirt over his head. At that point, being free of this internal war felt impossible. There was constant pressure in the front of my head and seeing clearly demanded a lot of effort.

Wendy and I looked at each other and agreed with deep conviction that this desire to be happy should and would be fulfilled. Yet, we had no clue how to begin. We lived like monks and worked like scientists – researching ourselves, questioning and dissecting every thought, delving deeply into our respective selves – while discovering how to "complete and delete" our painful stories. Years earlier, we could not imagine living for even one entire day without the haunting, heavy feelings of fear, doubt, and worry.

Now, years later, as we are writing this, we realize that that brief conversation left an indelible impression on us both and planted the seeds of the system you are now reading. These seeds now have matured as we've cracked the code to happiness, and the haunting clouds of doubts are no more.

As a result of our soul-searching quest, we excavated and unearthed a complete and powerful system for choosing happiness and eliminating all doubts and worries in your life. We have worked out the kinks, so you can implement this system instantly. If we can pull ourselves out of our dungeons, like the Mines of Moria in *The Lord of the Rings,* and turn our lives around, you can do it too!

Now, the secrets to being *In Love Forever* are revealed.

Introduction

You may be saying, *"In Love Forever?* Seriously? There's no way. How can I be in love forever when I can't even remember what passion feels like? How can people make such claims? No one can really be *In Love Forever?* I mean, if we could, we'd all just do it, right?"

Since most romantic movies end and leave us wondering what happened to the pretty couple walking off into the sunset, that's where this book begins. We'll openly share with you how to live joyously after the sunset for years to come. This book will transform your love life, so you can live passionately and be *In Love Forever.* Here, we will generously reveal our secrets with you to help you clear out the painful circumstances, so you can create the relationship of your dreams. And each chapter ends with fun suggestions to make your dreams a reality.

Whether you are single or in a relationship, this book will lead you on a journey. The material is organized into bite-sized pieces, so you can easily and safely transform your relationship during a 90-day journey. We've even included suggestions at the end of each chapter summary, which you can focus on and follow for the next 10 days. These suggestions are meant to be continued throughout your life, but there's no pressure to follow this timeline. Go through the book at your own pace, but read the chapters in order to ensure old worn-out patterns or issues are cleared and replaced with a renewed and revitalized heart-centered relationship.

As you and your partner utilize the tools in this book, you are going to transform yourself and your relationship like never before – quickly and consistently. The arguing, pain, fear, distrust, disconnection, and lack of communication will evolve into a deeper connection between the two of you as you become more intimate emotionally. Your sensuality and lovemaking will be renewed along with an expanded spiritual connection.

Most journeys begin by taking a leap of faith and that first step. We are excited to assist you with transforming those familiar negative patterns of fear, anger, and jealousy, so they will stop destroying your passion for life and your relationship.

Being *In Love Forever* isn't difficult; it is simply new! Similarly, having a joyous, juicy, intimate, sustainable relationship isn't difficult either; it is simply new, as well!

What is so desirable or sexy about being fearful, angry, and unhappy? Do these offer any positive health benefits? When you worry, do you feel attractive or full of energy? Most of us *do* want to be genuinely happy all the time, but how do we get there?

Do you realize how powerful your choice is? Being *In Love Forever* is a choice. Do outside circumstances influence your choice to feel loving and happy in your relationship, your work, and in your family? For example, does the mirror determine how beautiful you look and feel? How about the amount of money in your bank account or how well your kids do in school? Or is your happiness based on how you choose to *respond* to these circumstances, whether things are going your way or not? In our work with countless couples and singles throughout the past 20 years, we find that most men and women allow *circumstances* to determine how happy and relationship-fulfilled they are.

Do not mistake us here: The genuine source of your happiness *cannot* be attached to your husband, your mother, your children, or your finances! Your genuine source of happiness lies *within* you. *It's your choice that determines the quality of life that you live.*

11

Now, we completely understand that you may feel hesitant as well as excited about transforming your life. Our suggestion: do not hesitate! Jump in with both feet, your whole heart, and a clear head ... just go for it! Begin now because, in our professional experience and opinion, there really isn't anything holding you back except your negative thoughts, doubts, fears, and frustration!

In Love Forever reveals the secrets to turning your pain into a partnership, relationship, and life you've dreamed about having. This step-by-step system will guide and show you how to easily communicate like never before and how to clear out pain and secrets in a supported manner together. You will feel a deeper, honest, and more joyous, juicy heart connection with your partner *no matter your circumstances*. And you will discover how fears, worries, and insecurities are the best thing that could happen to you.

Whatever has led you to this material indicates that you are ready to experience a more satisfied life, no longer negatively affected by doubts, fears, burdens, and fighting. Your professional and personal life will benefit from this 7 secret system, and your relationship will be renewed, refreshed, and revitalized. You may be surprised to find that you won't ever feel alone again as your connection and feeling of God/Source/Divine unmistakably evolves, and you both become beacons of joy for other couples and families.

If you're ready, let's get to work.

Would knowing how to create a juicy level of happiness, at will, anytime, anywhere, no matter what's going on in your life, positively impact your life? Would knowing how to create such an ecstatic feeling interest you? If your answer is yes, instead of judging life, you will learn to create happiness from the inside, appreciate the essence of life, ignite the fire and creative life force within yourself, and enjoy a deeper connection with your partner.

In the movie, *Meet Joe Black,* Brad Pitt ("Joe," who is the angel of death) and Jeffrey Tambor ("Quince") discuss love and its beauty and depth.

Joe

But Allison loves you?

Quince

(short, deep, guttural cry)

Joe

How do you know?

Quince

Because she knows the worst thing about me, and it's okay.

Joe

What is it?

Quince

No, it's not one thing. It's just an idea, Joe. It's just ... like, you know each other's secrets ... your deepest, darkest secrets.

Joe

Deepest, darkest secrets.

Quince

Yeah, and then you're free.

Joe

Free?

Quince

You're free! You're free to love each other. Completely. Totally. No fear. There's nothing that you don't know about each other, and it's okay.

We are about to pull back the curtain and provide you with many powerful tools and real life examples in an easy-to-use interactive style, showing you how being *In Love Forever* is attainable. These 7 secrets will guide you in bite-sized chunks to end any painful memories that you carry, leading you towards joy and success. Here we will show you an exciting new model for creating a joyful, juicy, and intimate relationship.

Choosing to be *In Love Forever* is in your hands. As William Shakespeare so eloquently wrote, *"The choices you make dictate the life you lead. To thine ownself be true."* A relationship is made up of two individuals, each having the power to *choose* to be happy or unhappy at any given moment. In the blink of an eye, you can influence each other, positively or negatively.

All your dreams are waiting.

We realize that manufacturing happiness takes sincere desire and dedication. The more you desire to transform yourself, the quicker the progress will be. Consider it like training as if you were preparing yourself to climb the Rocky Mountains. As you ascend into more happiness the views become more beautiful, yet the air thins, which makes the rest of the climb more challenging. However, if your desire is to be happy and to constantly make course corrections, you will reach your summit of joyous grandeur.

This idea of staying on course to reach your goals is similar to a pilot flying a commercial jet from LA to NY. Statistics show that 95 percent of the time the plane is traveling off course, thus the pilot is constantly course correcting to land the plane precisely at the airport.

Happiness is available to you this very second. You just need to choose it...allow it ... and discontinue doubting yourself and your ability to live your dreams.

Innovation is awaiting you once you choose to put the weapons of self-doubt and harshness down. You are actualizing your individual and relationship potential. Instead of just treading water, you will literally feel as if you're "above the clouds," living in the world but not of it. As you clear your doubts and fears and direct your life, you will have the time and financial success to craft your days and your relationship in the most delightful ways.

So, let's begin being *In Love Forever.*

Chapter 1

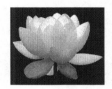

Secret 1a – Let's Get Real

"Anything will give up its secrets if you love it enough. Not only have I found that when I talk to the little flower or to the little peanut they will give up their secrets, but I have found that when I silently commune with people they give up their secrets also – if you love them enough."

~ George Washington Carver

Being transparent is one of the most important steps in the quest to being *In Love Forever.* First, let's have fun enhancing the level of transparency between you and your partner. This will begin to transform any difficulties you are presently experiencing, release any pains or hurts, and birth a deeper intimacy of joy in your relationship. Sounds great. "Yet, how do you to do this?" First, turn off your cell phones, toss aside the brief cases and diaper bags, and yank off your proverbial coats of armor from your busy day. Strip yourself completely naked of your 'role du jour.' Over time we tend to build a thick fortress around our hearts, denying our own truth and our power by lying, cheating, and hiding from ourselves and our partners.

If you're having difficulty communicating with your husband, your wife, your kids, or your boss, you cannot afford *not* to do this! Think of it like this: You occasionally clear out old files on your computer, right? When your computer has an overload of unneeded, extraneous files, the system runs as slow as molasses and creates massive frustration. When we delete these files, the computer runs much more efficiently. Well, it's the same with humans. When we clear out old, hidden, secretive stories and lies, we literally lighten up, have more energy, and feel an expansion of love in our hearts.

Let's begin. Schedule a night free from distractions. Turn off all electronics: phones, TV, computer, etc. Order-in delicious comfort food, and be sure your kids are quiet and/or well occupied for the evening.

You'll answer a set of questions that will clear any doubts, fears, and insecurities you've been carrying – the heavy baggage – throughout your life. Enjoy being nakedly honest. The more honest you are, the more baggage you'll discard. Be compassionate, gentle, and kind to yourself. Approach this as an adventure, a discovery. It's exhilarating to learn new characteristics and aspects about your self and your partner.

Self-Inquiry Questionnaire

Answer the questions **by yourself.** *Do not* share your answers with your partner just yet. It is essential to keep this information to yourself until you have read Chapter 2 (*What You Don't Know Will Hurt You*), which will prepare you to appropriately share and listen to your partner's answers. If you are single, answer the questions to the best of your ability, and if you're comfortable sharing your answers with a trusted friend or family member, do so. (They may wish to answer these questions as well and share them with you.) Before every question, say "On a scale from 1–10 ..." (i.e. On a scale from 1–10, rate your level of happiness today).

*(If the questions are too emotionally charged for you, and you feel you can't answer them, stop. Take a short break to compose yourself. When you come back to the questions, if they are still too difficult to answer, please immediately seek out a professional relationship coach or therapist who can assist you through whatever the issue/issues are and return to answering the questions only after you feel more comfortable and ready to proceed.)

RATE THE QUESTIONS ON A SCALE OF 1–10.
(10 BEING THE HIGHEST, 1 BEING THE LEAST)

1.

a. Rate your level of happiness today.

_____

b. Rate your level of happiness when you were a child.

_____

2.

a. Rate the level of happiness in your parent's relationship.

_____

b. How well do /did your parents deal with their emotions?

_____

c. Rate how your happiness as a youth was influenced by the level of happiness in your parents' relationship.

_____

d. How physically intimate are /were your parents?

_____

e. How emotionally and spiritually intimate are /were your parents?

_____

3.

a. How aware are you of your inner challenges, such as your fears, doubts, insecurities, needs, etc.?

_____

b. Rate how often you communicate about these inner challenges with someone close to you, like your partner, close friend, or a coach.

_____

c. How comfortable do you feel talking about your feelings, emotions, frustrations, worries, joys, etc.?

_____

4.

a. How aware are you of your dreams and goals in life?

_____

b. How well have you communicated your dreams to your partner, close friend, or coach?

_____

c. How well are your dreams supported by your partner, close friend, or coach?

_____

d. To what degree are you living your dreams and reaching your goals?

_____

5.

a. When your most intense doubt or fear arises, how often are you able to completely transform the intense "heavy, blackened feelings" within five minutes or less?

_____

b. When you feel nervous, angry, drained, depressed, numb, or sad, how well are you able to contain and work out these feelings without having a negative effect on your partner, your family, co-workers, and friends?

_____

6.

a. How often do you worry about your body looking right? i.e. weight, age, and level of attractiveness.

_____

b. Rate how great you feel about yourself when looking in the mirror.

_____

7.

a. As you're getting ready for a romantic night out, <u>with lovemaking on your mind for the end of the evening,</u> how often does the evening get ruined by negative "self talk," such as, "We don't have the money to go out," or "I'm not as thin and beautiful/handsome as I want to be?"

_____

b. How often do you share those negative thoughts with your partner?

_____

c. How comfortable do you feel talking about your feelings, emotions, frustrations, worries, joys, etc. with your partner?

_____

d. How often do you make love before you go out for dinner or a romantic evening?

_____

8. Rate your level of physical discomfort /pain.

_____

9.

a. How often do you worry about money and your ability to provide financially for yourself and your family?

_____

b. How much are you creating your livelihood from your talents and gifts?

_____

10.

a. Rate yourself in terms of being an alcoholic, drug addict, workaholic, food or sex addict, war veteran, sexual abuse survivor, or other.

_____

b. How much are you able to imagine that any and all emotional trauma you've experienced will no longer negatively affect you?

_____

SUBTOTAL SCORE – SECTION A: _____

*(Next, if you are single and have experienced a relationship break-up or divorce, answer the following questions from your past experience. Reflecting about the past may bring up feelings but keep breathing. The point of this inquiry is to gain vital insights about yourself. It will enable you to create the luscious, intimate relationship of your dreams.)

RATE THE QUESTIONS ON A SCALE OF 1–10.
(10 BEING THE HIGHEST, 1 BEING THE LEAST)

1. Rate the level of romance in your relationship now.

_____

2. How satisfied are you with lovemaking with your partner?

_____

3. How important is lovemaking with your partner?

_____

4. Does your desire to make love ever wane when you are worried?

_____

5.

a. How much does your partner know about what pleases you?

_____

b. Does your partner take the time to please you?

_____

6.

a. How present are you during lovemaking with your partner?

_____

b. Do you ever fantasize about making love with someone other than your partner?

_____

c. Are you ever preoccupied with other worries or distractions that take you away from the lovemaking experience?

7.

a. How often have you secretly looked at naked men or women in magazines or on the Internet while in your present relationship?

b. How comfortable do you feel discussing the "topic of sex" with your partner?

8.

a. How well do you work with your partner as a team?

b. Rate the amount of quality time you spend with your partner and your family.

SUBTOTAL SCORE – SECTION B: _____

If you are single, answer the following yes or no questions.

1. Do you have any unresolved issues about a divorce or break-up in your life now? Yes____ No____

2.

a. Have you ever been with a partner unwilling to commit to the relationship?   Yes_____ No_____

b. Have you ever been in a relationship with someone who is married?   Yes_____ No_____

c. Are you completely ready to commit to a healthy relationship?   Yes_____ No_____

Whether you are in a relationship or presently single, answering the following questions will bring deeper insight into your life.

Explain any negative thoughts you have about your body.

_____
_____
_____
_____
_____
_____
_____
_____

Explain any challenges you feel when talking about your feelings, emotions, worries, frustrations, joy, etc. with your partner.

_____
_____
_____
_____
_____
_____
_____
_____
_____

What are your dreams and goals?

_____
_____
_____
_____
_____
_____
_____
_____

Have you written your dreams and goals down before?   Yes_____ No_____

If so, do you revisit them and update them daily/monthly/semi-annually?   Yes_____ No_____

How can your partner improve when supporting and inspiring you to realize your dreams and goals?

_____

_____

_____

_____

_____

_____

_____

_____

What unresolved issues are still present in your life from prior relationships?

_____

_____

_____

_____

_____

_____

_____

_____

_____

_____

Who are your exemplifying "loving relationship" heroes? Why?

_____
_____
_____
_____
_____
_____
_____
_____
_____
_____

Reflecting on your prior relationship(s), what characteristics would you choose to change about yourself in order to experience your desired relationship now?

_____
_____
_____
_____
_____
_____
_____
_____

TABULATE YOUR SCORE BY ADDING
THE A AND B SUBTOTALS

SUBTOTAL A _____

SUBTOTAL B _____

TOTAL SCORE _____

Congratulations on finishing the questionnaire! Now that you've tabulated Sections A and B and have your total score, let's find out what it means. Find the score range that matches your total.

If your score is:

400–310. Your score indicates that you and your partner are very compatible, communicate clearly with each other, and take deep care to maintain a juicy, loving relationship. Continue to work to deepen your intimacy, creating a lifetime of being in love. Take time to acknowledge where you are and where you want to go in your relationship.

309–209. Your score reveals that you and your partner are feeling like your relationship is strong, but there is room for a tune-up in some areas to help your relationship continue to ascend in a caring, loving manner. It's important that you and your partner communicate transparently regarding the areas which you feel need improvement, so you can begin to transform them. You might benefit from working with a relationship coach or therapist to quickly smooth out the rough edges in the relationship. Take time to acknowledge where you are and where you want to go in your relationship.

208 or less. Your score suggests that there are several areas in your relationship that are causing friction. Honest, transparent, heart-to-heart communication awaits you and will help you explore and transform any and all tension between you. Do you have the desire to improve your relationship? If so, encourage each other to take action immediately. The good news is there are a lot of qualified relationship coaches/therapists to assist you both in safely transforming your relationship. Put your focus on where you want to go. As you turn around these present challenges, you will feel more joyous in your life and in your relationship. Take time to acknowledge where you are and where you want to go in your relationship.

Partner Questionnaire

Now that you have completed the first step, take a break. When you are ready to come back, answer all the questions again, but this time answer from the perspective of your partner. For example, rate your **partner's** level of happiness today.

Again, we cannot stress enough the importance of approaching these questions with a sense of discovery, joy, and adventure.

Congratulations on completing the steps! Here's the intent: anyone who reads this material will absolutely succeed in reaching his or her goals and dreams. Your responses will be very fruitful as we continue. You may now want to wrap yourself up in a blanket with a cup of tea, take a soothing bath or hot tub, or perhaps take a walk outside.

Remember, as airplanes climb up to new heights, they often go through turbulence. This deep inquiry may be very new for you, and you may find yourself falling asleep, crying, or even getting angry while answering the questions. Allow your feelings to surface.

It's important to remember that the more you put yourself into this material, the more you and your partner will get out of it. As you choose to change, you will be forging a new path of massive positive change in our world, where man and woman joyously come together like never before. We thank you very much for your courage!

Once you have both finished writing down your answers, you can share your answers but ONLY about yourself. DO NOT share what you wrote about your partner until you have BOTH completely read Chapter 2.

Listen to Your Love or Wedding Song Together

Do you have a love or wedding song for your relationship? If so, this might be a good time to listen to it and look into each other's eyes and say, "Whatever challenges we are experiencing, I choose to figure them out and deepen my love for you starting now." (Check out Appendix E for a list of Love Songs.)

Next, in Chapter 2, we have created extremely effective, time-tested communication tools – which we developed over many years – to help you learn how to effectively and safely share answers with your partner.

The Power of Commitment

"Until one is committed, there is hesitancy, the chance to draw back, always ineffectiveness. Concerning all acts of initiative & creation, there is one elementary truth, the ignorance of which kills countless ideas and splendid plans:

"That the moment one definitely commits oneself, then providence moves too. All sorts of things begin to happen that would never otherwise have occurred.

"A whole stream of events issues from the decision, raising in one's favor all manner of unforeseen incidents, meetings & material assistance, which no man could have dreamt would have come his way.

"I have a profound respect for one of Goethe's couplets:

'Whatever you can do or
dream you can, begin it.

Boldness has genius,
power, & magic in it.'

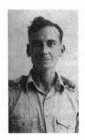

*Quoted from the book
"The Scottish Himalayan Expedition, 1951"
by William H. Murray (1913-1996)*

CHAPTER SUMMARY POINTS

*"He looked at her the way all women
want to be looked at by a man."*

~ F. Scott Fitzgerald, <u>The Great Gatsby</u>

- Although it can be intense, cultivate an approach of discovery while talking about your feelings with your partner or trusted friend. Such honest, open talks will have a profound and positive impact on you and your partnership.

- You may go through turbulence answering these questions. Allow the feelings to surface as they are precious gems.

- Start noticing when/if you "bite" into the poisoned apple of fear. Begin to notice how your demeanor affects others around you.

- If you have experienced a divorce or break-up, this is a great time to clear up any and all unresolved feelings and to move forward.

- If you are attracting partners who are unwilling to commit, take note. It takes two to tango. There's probably room in the area of commitment for you to transform as well.

- Relinquish complacency and take a quantum leap.

- Watch the films *Fireproof* and *Meet the Fockers*.

- Listen to your love or wedding song and declare your choice to transform the present challenges into more joy, love and nurturance in your relationship. For a list of love songs, look at Appendix E.

- 90 day journey: Clear out personal past histories that are blocking your joy in the present (i.e. trust issues and feeling passionate).

Click the link below or go online to access our Top 10 Romantic Movies of all time at InLoveForeverBook.com

Chapter 2

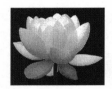

Secret 1b – What You Don't Know Will Hurt You

"When all your desires are distilled;
You will cast just two votes:
To love more and be happy."

~ Rumi

Welcome back!

Let's take the next step on this adventure toward discovery. By now, you have completed the questions in Chapter 1. If not, please do so. Before entering into the communication exercises with your partner or trusted friend, you need to complete these questions. In this chapter, you will discover effective communication tools and innovative concepts which can be instantly integrated into your life; tools that we and countless other couples have time-tested through our coaching programs. You will discover real life examples of how these tools have positively impacted our lives and the lives of other couples.

Using these tools will help clear out any built up feelings of hurt or resentment from childhood to present day, along with any insecurities, secrets, depressive thoughts, etc. and invigorate your passion and sense of satisfaction with your life – enhancing emotional intimacy with yourself, your partner, family, and friends and creating a deeper connection with the Divine.

Because communication is crucial, we will spend quite a bit of time preparing you for these exercises. Incorporating these communication tools and concepts into your lives will help you build a vital foundation for the breakthrough information to come in forthcoming chapters.

Let Go of Blame

Be careful not to go into these talks with blame in your back pocket. For example, you may feel, "Finally, I am getting a chance to really speak my mind to my partner and get back at her, so that she can begin to change."

Caution! You both need to enter into this communication experience by taking full responsibility for your life, your thoughts, and all of your choices. Remember to manage your reactions and feelings. Remember, as well, you can only change yourself, so change yourself in a way that will inspire your partner or partner-to-be to do the same.

Why Delve So Deep?

There's a treasure chest of unlimited possibilities deep inside of you. In order to discover them, you need to clear out all that's blocking your grandness. You may be in emotional discomfort or pain. Instead of turning away from it, snuggle up to it. Here you will learn to go through the pain and transform it. Let's face it: Pain is one of humanity's greatest motivators for transformation. Rather than holding in your feelings, which lead to disease, follow the advice offered in these great song lyrics from John Mayer's song, "Say":

> *Say what you need to say... You better know that in the end / It's better to say too much / Than never to say what you need to say again... Even*

if your hands are shakin' / And your faith is broken / Even as the eyes are closin' / Do it with a heart wide open...Say what you need to say."

Remember, as you are sharing your answers with each other, emotions may flare up at times. This is to be expected, so prepare for it and allow yourself to express intensity as it comes. Don't worry about being perfect at implementing these communication tools immediately. Give yourselves the gift of patience.

As you begin the process, you may feel worse as the pot gets stirred up. Like when a river is being dredged, initially the water looks very murky, even dirtier than before. But gradually the water will clear up, and the river will become healthier and livelier. So begin to dredge out your crud! Step by step, you will become happier and will be able to put an end to your old, painful stories.

Keep this in mind as well: While you may present a positive happy image on the outside, you may be an emotional mess on the inside. These deep, painful experiences in your heart tend to cycle and recycle within you. You may have found ways to push these painful issues down in the past. Perhaps, you take drugs, have sex, or drink alcohol to numb the painful memories. Or perhaps you overwork to keep these stories deep down inside of you. None of these approaches benefits you in the long run, so it's time to open up and lighten your load!

What Do We Talk About?

Essentially, the purpose is to share feelings and stories that are bugging you. We all have stories that we may hold in; dreams that have been buried alive; unresolved situations that have occurred over the years between us and our partners. Perhaps there are incidents with your family or past traumas that continue to haunt you, or crushes or attractions that you had as a youth or even as an adult which still rise to the surface. Admitting these things to your partner can be very freeing.

Some of these stories may be familiar to your partner if you've shared them over the years, or perhaps he or she has never heard them at all. There could be stories deep inside of you that no one has ever heard. Now's the time to let them all out!

Don't be afraid to expose your most grungy and embarrassing truths either, otherwise known as your "cheats in the sheets." While the phrase may sound peculiar, your honesty will set you free.

Open up and talk with each other about how you feel about your intimate expression. Are you pleasing each other? Are there ways which you can please your partner more (and yourself as well). Guys, if you have issues about your penis size, this is a great moment to discuss this and get the concern off your chest. You may be surprised to learn that your partner is satisfied with your penis size. With the burden lifted, you can really enjoy what you've got.

Our Personal Story

In the heat of our difficulties while on the brink of divorce, we made a commitment to change. We took a week out of our lives, ordered food, turned off our phones, and shut out all the distractions and just talked ... all day and all night about anything and everything.

We both remember that at the beginning it was quite scary because we didn't feel we had anything much to say to each other. Yet we had made a commitment to stay in this process for one week — no matter what. But once we started, we didn't want to shut up. We were having so much fun!

We talked about a lot of things that were uncomfortable and continued to stir the pot, so to speak. We looked at ourselves and each other in the mirror naked and talked about the shame and likes and dislikes we felt about our bodies. These were very intimate, endearing moments.

At that point we decided to lift the sheets and share about everything, revealing our "cheats in the sheets." And we realized something amazing. We had unspoken agreements between us to never go to certain places that might stir up uncomfortable feelings. Sexuality was one of those areas; a big overloaded file that was dragging us both down. Initially we were afraid to go there, so we tested the waters with our baby toes.

We discovered that we had different attractions or fantasies about certain people, but we never talked about them because it was too scary or embarrassing. We even spoke about our first intimate encounter together, admitting how we both had an image that our naked bodies would look different than they did. Cary expressed that he hoped that first night was going to be a bit wilder.

When we started to talk about these issues, we anticipated a volcano-sized fight would erupt. Instead, once we started to open up and share our fantasies, we started to crack up at ourselves and each other. We were exploding with laughter. Actually, we felt relieved to finally be so honest.

The result of these talks wasn't about going out and getting a facelift or a tummy tuck or taking supplements for male enhancement. Rather, it was about coming to a place of acceptance and joy for our bodies. We felt a deepening trust and light-heartedness beginning to grow between us.

Personally speaking, that week made such a huge change in our relationship and brought us together like never before, and now there is nothing that we cannot talk about, nothing that would embarrass or shock us.

The depth of our honesty from that week, together with the power of these communication tools, gave us a solid foundation and the strength to overcome our difficulties together. As a result, our relationship continues to flourish today.

If we got that "lovin' feeling" back, then you can, too!

Communication Tools

A. Sandbox Talk

B. Transcribing

C. Capsule

Ground Rules

- Respect each other
- No cross talking

Once you begin, be mindful not to interrupt your partner. Feelings may come up, but please do not "cross talk" or interrupt one another. At times, as a listener, your buttons will be pushed, and you might feel tempted to lash out and defend yourself. The hairs on your arms may stand up. You may feel that your partner is picking on you, or that you have done something wrong. Try inwardly repeating the following phrases: "That's a truth," or "That's one way to look at it." This will help you stay neutral; so, clear your feelings and remain silent.

Do not "yeah-but" the speaker's truths. Rather, hear your partner with a caring heart, and know that he or she is expressing something very important. You do not have to agree with his or her truth, but breathe into it and keep listening.

The more that you can listen attentively to your partner while holding a neutral space, the easier it will be for him or her to let down his or her guard and then truly listen to you as well without a pre-set agenda.

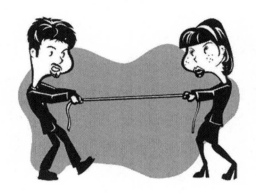

At times, you will "bite" into being right. OH, THE PRICE OF BEING RIGHT! Remember to breathe, laugh, whistle, blow bubbles, and let go of your end of the rope ... do whatever it takes to reduce the unhappy intensity. After all, what's so sexy about being right and bitter? So, embrace being wrong for a change!

Your partner may be calling you on a behavior that it would benefit you greatly to change. Sometimes this is a big "OUCH" to hear but hang in there. It is a blessing to have a mirror to help you let go of limiting behaviors, so you don't stagnate in complacency. By sharing at such a core level, you will build new levels of trust and intimacy together.

- **Use "I" statements.**

  For example, try saying, "I feel frustrated when you did/said this..." instead of, "You pissed me off when you did/said this ..."

- **Create a time frame for each other.**

  You may want to start out with five minutes for each person. Believe it or not, that's a long time to talk. After that, try 15 minutes of uninterrupted speech.

  During the designated time, the speaker can say anything. The other person is just listening. The listener should also act as the timekeeper and needs to be clear and kind when letting the speaker know when two minutes are left. The speaker shouldn't worry if he or she does not express everything at once. There will be plenty of time to talk again.

- **Never damage anything or be hurtful to each other.**

  Remember not to criticize someone's character faults, but rather focus on the behavior. You may not agree with your partner's truths, but make a great effort not to crush him or her either.

- **Neither partner is allowed to leave the room until the exercise is completed.**

- **Become a neutral listener.**

As a listener, remember constantly that what your partner is sharing is about <u>him or her</u>, not about you. You are your partner's mirror, a neutral listener. Stay present and stay caring.

A. Sandbox Talk

Purpose

When you take the time to clear out the old laundry, so to speak, you give yourself a chance to build a greater level of intimacy. Try to create a relaxed format, so you can talk about vulnerable issues. This is a good beginning tool to practice opening up to one another and can be used on an ongoing basis.

Level of Intensity - Light to moderate

Creating the Context

A *Sandbox Talk* is designed to help you call forth a safe space to open up, like two kids playing together in a sandbox, making fun magical things like best buddies do. A let-your-hair-down approach is what we want to create here.

Sandbox Talks can be a lot of fun because they keep getting deeper the longer you engage in them. You may want to grab a good cup of coffee or tea while you are talking.

Did you ever have a time with your partner when you just wanted to talk and talk and talk? A time spent getting to know each other's dreams and visions while wanting to learn everything about each other? *Sandbox Talks* can rekindle that type of excitement and get your creative juices flowing again.

What is the recommended amount of time to spend on the *Sandbox Talk*?

Many of us are very bottled up and could highly benefit initially from a concentrated amount of time to "defrost." The more time you can reserve for this, the quicker your results will be.

You may need time to rest and simply unwind from an extremely demanding and busy life. But don't worry, you will know what amount of time is right for your situation.

If you have kids, consider arranging a babysitter for a date night on a regular basis. No matter how busy you are, make it a priority to talk for at least 20–30 minutes every day (i.e. before the day begins or at the end of the day).

DO NOT PUT YOUR LIVES OFF. ACT NOW.

EVERY SECOND IS PRECIOUS!

Know that everyone in your family will highly benefit from the time you spend creating a new juicy level of intimacy. When you value this intimacy with yourself and your partner, then miracles will come to support you both in your life and will provide you with the necessary time and resources you may need. And always, always, remember to ask for help!

Example:

Robert and Ann have two children: one in the fifth grade and one in the seventh. Ann would like to gift the kids with a two-week summer camp of their interest: soccer and baseball.

Every time Ann brings the subject up with Robert they end up in a fight, both blaming each other for their frustrations. Ann feels frustrated that they can never get past Robert's beliefs about their financial situation. Over the years, Robert has been the main income earner for the family, and his present income is not enough to pay for these camps with all the other expenses the family incurs.

So Ann calls for a Sandbox Talk. She begins by acknowledging that Robert has not been interested in the idea of the summer camps because he feels they can't afford the cost. She notes that Robert does see the value in the kids going to the camps, yet he has been triggered by Ann's enthusiasm to invest in the kids' creative endeavors.

Even though they have a line of credit available to them with low interest rates, Robert does not want to use this for funding the camps. He is afraid to go into further debt. Ann utilizes the Sandbox Talk to impress upon Robert that this would be a very valuable experience for the children, and, in time, they would find ways to pay for the camps.

This talk opens an old wound of Robert's belief systems about financially being supported. As the talk continues, he begins to realize his frustrations and anger toward Ann for not bringing in more income throughout their married years.

Ann painfully realizes how she has suppressed her own desires to create a job that she loves, which can be financially successful. Over the years, she struggled to believe in her ability to start a new business of her own, so she opted to work for others, doing more secure part-time jobs.

They realize, together, that they have been isolating themselves from each other and hiding in the dark corners of their fears, afraid to deal with the issue of financial insecurity. It had been too scary for them to address their individual underlying fears about being supported. They commit to writing out their goals and dreams and to working intensively together over several months to get to and clear out the root of their fears.

Much of their attention had been focused on the children; therefore, the quality of their intimacy suffered. They now see the value in investing in themselves and the relationship and getting intimate and juicy again. They acknowledge their trepidation toward change, but the love they feel for their two *children and each other gives them the reason to jump into the unknown and work it out as they go.*

Through this deepening process with his wife, Robert decides that he really wants to gift his children with the opportunity to go to camp. He sees in a funny way now that his fear of money has been holding his own creativity back as well and realizes that this work with his wife is opening doors for him to grow professionally and financially. From being initially resistant and afraid to open up to his wife, he now is excited as he is experiencing positive results.

B. Transcribing

Purpose

This method is very useful when you want your partner to understand exactly what it is that you are trying to say. In this approach, the listener becomes a transcriber. This type of communication is referred to as call and response.

Basically, one person speaks and says an idea in short snippets, and the listener repeats back (or "mirrors") exactly what the speaker says. The listener doesn't add any of his or her ideas. It's not necessary that you repeat the ideas back to your partner word for word; however, the essence should be impeccably accurate.

Once you've repeated the ideas to your partner, check back with him or her by asking, "Did I get that right?" If the speaker feels that the response was not accurate, then he or she will say, "No, what I meant was ..."

Then the listener should repeat the accurate information back and ask, "Is there more?" This dialogue should continue back and forth until the speaker feels that he or she has expressed everything completely.

After mirroring back precisely what the speaker had to say, the listener then acknowledges what was said. For example, "Hearing what you have said, I can now understand why you feel the way you do."

Level of Intensity - Medium to medium hot

Creating the Context

Transcribing is a fabulous way to sharpen your listening skills, so you are really able to hear the important information your partner wishes to share. You may feel that you are expressing yourself very clearly and get frustrated that your partner does not seem to understand what you are saying. This tool will sharpen your mind and open your hearts to each other and can be very useful throughout your lives. *Transcribing* is more specialized and used less frequently than the *Sandbox Talk*.

What Do We Talk About?

Feel free to discuss any issue that you feel is important to share with your partner.

Example:

David feels frustrated that he can't seem to get his point across to Jennifer, as she keeps interrupting him with comments that are not related to what he is saying. David, therefore, asks for a transcribing session, so he can express himself uninterruptedly. Jennifer repeats back to him the essence of what he's saying to make sure she clearly understands what he is communicating to her.

David: "I feel so frustrated that you are not hearing what I'm saying."

Jennifer: "You feel so frustrated when I am not hearing what you are saying."

David: "When I speak, I feel like your head is in the clouds."

Jennifer: "When you speak, you feel like my head is in the clouds."

David: "This has happened many times lately."

Jennifer: "This has happened many times lately."

David: "When I communicate an idea to you, you often answer me with something totally different than what I said."

Jennifer: "When you talk to me, I often respond back to you with something totally different."

David: "I am very angry and frustrated. Where is my woman?"

Jennifer: "You are very frustrated and angry. You are wondering where your woman is."

David: "I feel afraid when you are not present with me. I feel I'm losing you."

Jennifer: "You feel afraid when I am not present with you. You feel like you are losing me."

David: "Please listen to me and wait until I'm finished before you add your comments."

Jennifer: "You're requesting that I listen to you and hold back my comments until you are finished. Did I get that right?"

David: "Yes."

Jennifer: "Is there more?"

David: "No, my thoughts are complete."

Jennifer: "I can understand why you have felt frustrated, and I will sincerely sharpen my listening skills when you speak to me."

David: "Thank you. I really appreciate that."

C. Capsule

Purpose

The purpose of the capsule is to release very intense repressed feelings, such as angst, anger, fear, frustrations, and doubt. Impeccable honesty is recommended in order to get in touch with primal feelings. Speakers should not worry about feeling inhibited or being kind or nice while releasing deep-seated unresolved issues about their partners, someone else, or some frustrating situation or pattern.

This is a place where you can vent. Let it rip! Express the things that really piss you both off about each other. You may be very emotional and initially blame the other person. This is acceptable here because we are intending to purge repressed feelings. Please follow the steps implicitly. **To achieve the best results,** make a copy if needed, of this section and the summary points to have with you when you utilize this technique.

At the end, the listener acknowledges the speaker's truths.

Level of Intensity - Hot to very hot

Creating the Context

It is up to the individual to call a *Capsule* session. It is a spontaneous occurrence when the feelings are unbearable, and they need to be expressed immediately. The listener must be very strong while maintaining a neutral space.

Before beginning, it's important that each of you take a moment and envision sitting in your own actual capsule, perhaps built by NASA. The idea is that the listener is in his or her own bubble and is not allowing the intense feelings of the speaker to affect him or her.

The listener gives the speaker the space to express very intense feelings. As previously stated, the listener may want to repeat silently to himself or herself, "That's a truth," or "That's one way to look at it."

Remember to not cross talk or leave the room no matter how intense the feelings get.

It is important for the listener to not take these feelings personally, although it can feel intensely personal. As the feelings are being released, the speaker must remember that although he or she may be feeling very disturbed by something his or her partner or someone else did, ultimately he or she must own the feelings.

What is the recommended amount of time to spend on *The Capsule?*

There is no rule regarding how long the intervals should be, but you may want to limit them to 10–15 minute segments. Again, these sessions are very different than the *Sandbox Talks,* as they are spontaneous and intermittent, depending on the level and intensity of the feelings.

What Do We Talk About?

Whatever is concerning you at the moment.

Example:

Paul expresses to Maria his long held-in frustrations about how cold and controlling she has become.

"I'm so angry with you that you're not emotionally available for me. You are so controlling! We used to have great sex together. What happened?

"It's been so long. I am still attracted to you, strange as that may seem, and it pisses me off that you seem to be so uninterested in having sex with me.

"This angers me so much. It's like a game you're playing with me. At the beginning of our relationship, you put it out to catch me. And catch me you did! But as time went on, you gave it out less and less.

"Well, whether it's right or wrong, I need to have sex. I want to have sex. And I want to find a way to reclaim that with us. But if we can't, I'm going to find someone else.

"In the last year or so, you have not even been pleasing me. You have made no effort to please me. So, what the hell are we together for? Can you answer me that question?

"And it really gets my blood boiling when I've overheard you man bashing with your girlfriends. Where's your heart? What do you care about anymore? Where are your feelings?

"I mean, don't you want to have sex anymore? Don't you miss it? Do you even care about me and what my feelings are? Lately, it just always seems to be that it's all about you, you, you, you. I'm sick and tired of it.

"We've got to have some massive change here, or this relationship is over!"

Maria responds after a long silence.

"I can really feel that you are upset. I am upset, too, and confused about what you are saying. I am committed to change and to working this out with you. I do care for you, and you are right."

Later on, Maria calls for a *Sandbox Talk* to share her insights about her lack of sexual desire. She begins to see that her pulling away from Paul sexually had nothing to do with a lack of attraction for him but was based on her own poor body image. They both agree that it's going to take some time to work this issue out, but they are very excited and hopeful to do so together. Please go to Chapter 3 to read an article on the power that your body image has in your life.

CHAPTER SUMMARY POINTS

*"So it's not gonna be easy. It's gonna be really hard.
We're gonna have to work at this every day, but I
want to do that because I want you. I want all
of you, forever, you and me, every day…"*

~ Noah, *The Notebook*

- Master the concept of listening and clearly expressing yourself. Open up and admit even the most embarrassing truths, and you will feel lighter.

- Every day, even for 10 minutes, utilize at least one of these tools with your partner or trusted friend.

- When communicating, remember not to cross talk. Always use "I" statements when you are expressing something important. Never leave the room during the communication sessions. The listener is the timekeeper.

- Take an inventory on a daily basis of your patterns of blame, criticism, and scrutiny of yourself, others, or the world.

- After you complete any of the communication sessions, remember to take a moment and appreciate each other.

- Be thirsty to continually learn something new about your partner!

- Watch the films *Defending Your Life, Rocky III, Children of a Lesser God and The American President.*

- 90-day journey: Improve your communication with your partner by being more clear and direct. Discontinue blaming. Deepen trust using the communication tools, Sandbox Talk, Transcribing, and Capsule.

Extra Bonus –

Answer a RELATIONSHIP QUESTIONNAIRE. This will give you insight and be an eye opener as to the present state of your union.

Click the link below or go online to access the Relationship Questionnaire at InLoveForeverBook.com.

Now is a good time to complete the questionnaire. Make two copies of the questionnaire as we'll remind you to complete it again at the end of the book to get a realistic sense of how much has transformed during the course of implementing these tools.

By integrating the tools in this book, the positive transformations will likely create permanent new patterns, and if any tweaking needs to happen in the future, you'll both sense this and be able to get back on the right track very quickly.

Chapter 3

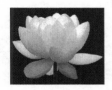

Secret 2 – Having Doubts Is the Best Thing For You

"The Constitution only gives people the right to pursue happiness. You have to catch it yourself."

~ Benjamin Franklin

Consider the word "doubt"

as a verb:

> *to be uncertain about; consider questionable or unlikely; hesitate to believe; to distrust; to fear; be apprehensive about; to be uncertain about something; to be undecided in opinion or belief*

as a noun:

> *a feeling of uncertainty about the truth, reality, or nature of something; distrust; fear; dread*

common synonyms:

> *distrust, mistrust, question, suspect*

related words:

> *disbelieve, discredit, negate, anxiety, concern, paranoia*

Examples:

> *I still have moments of doubt.*

> *I had a nagging doubt in the back of my mind.*

definitions from Merriam-Webster Dictionary

The information in this chapter is going to profoundly impact your life forever. In the previous chapters, we built a solid foundation for being *In Love Forever.* This next step is going to help you bring all of that information together.

Doubt Is Your Trainer – This important concept will help you turn your doubts inside out quickly. By doing this you will feel the doubts begin to disappear. As the heavy, darkened feelings transform, you will feel a renewed sense of joy and inspiration and a deeper connection with the Divine.

For far too long, so many of us have "bitten" into the doubts without knowing that there were other choices. What we mean by this is that we tend to believe that these thoughts, fears, and insecurities are true. For example, you may hear yourself thinking, "I'll never be supported. I am alone and exhausted as a single mom." This thought can take you down the well of despair. But there is another alternative, as you can see in the maps in the appendix, and this means slowing down that train of thought and starting to think or say, "No. I choose to stop 'biting.'" Then, say **the opposite,** "Help is on the way. I am surrounded by support. I have lots of friends. I'm not sure where the assistance will come from, yet I will keep pumping myself up with positive thoughts. I choose now to be completely supported, and I choose to create all of my dreams and desires effortlessly." Later in the chapter, the 5-step system will be detailed, and by following these simple steps, the negative effects of the doubts will end and your life will be forever transformed.

Doubt's purpose was never meant to take you down. The doubt is a reminder to pump up your dreams. In fact, the doubts are there to champion you. The doubt is your coach, your trainer, your fuel, your gatekeeper, your checkpoint, and it is monitoring you to make sure you get to where you want to go. Doubts are an incredible gift because they check to see how much you truly desire to create your visions, dreams, innovations, businesses, etc. while loving yourself and others.

"Doubt" Scrambled = To Bud

Like a lotus flower waiting to bud, there is beauty and power awaiting you, especially in your darkest and most limiting thoughts about yourself. People in the world have revered the lotus for many centuries. If you've ever smelled this flower, you may agree that the scent is indescribably beautiful. It is unique and special, and you, dear friend, are like a lotus flower just waiting to bud. We are all incredibly unique beings, and the world is waiting to experience your beautiful, sweet fragrance.

Turn Your Doubts Inside Out

It's time to reveal your original self. By thinking of your doubts in reverse, you will change your life forever! For example, if you hear in your head, "That's a ridiculous business idea. I'm not talented enough, not beautiful enough, etc. I'm never going to make enough money to support myself and my family," then take a moment to consider that things may not be as they appear. While you may feel like doubt is your worst enemy, truthfully, doubt is one of your best friends. When you realize this, you will never feel despair, depressed, or empty again.

Doubt persistently makes sure you follow your heart's yearnings; it cares deeply for your well-being, and it pushes you toward your desired finish line. Stop the doubt in its tracks. Accept what it says with a smile on your face and start putting in the opposite thought.

Often doubts occur at lightning speed, and, in the beginning when you're working to transform your doubts, you may very well "bite" into the "poisoned apple" before you even realize it. Perhaps you have "bitten" into the doubt that you can't make enough money. How does that make you feel? It feels pretty terrible, doesn't it? If you "bite" and find yourself spiraling downward, accept yourself. Recognize that you have "bitten" and then take responsibility for that choice. Climb out of the well, brush off the dirt, and start making new choices.

Recognizing the doubts as they arise is key. Ask yourself what they might be trying to tell you. What might their message be? How are you changing to fulfill your potential? Doubts have a purpose, but we never knew that their purpose was positive! Remember, no matter what the negative doubt was, the opposite is true, and the doubt is trying to get you to believe that, strengthen your resolve, and deepen your connection with Source / God / Divine. For example, in your head you might hear, "You are ugly." The doubt means that "you are beautiful," but you need to be aware of your thoughts and see how quickly you can turn that doubt around. Now that you understand this, when a doubt arises, you can get excited knowing that you are on the right path. The doubt is training you to become all that you are.

In the past, these negative statements may have taken you down emotionally, but that was never their intention. Who you are becoming is only temporarily restrained by these doubts. So, it's important to see that doubt has never been there to try to suppress you or make you feel depressed or anxious about your talents or purpose. These doubts are your trainers. They are trying to cheer you on toward reaching your goals. You may say, "What are you talking about? How could such negative voices actually have my best interests in mind?"

Learn to decode the doubts. Whatever the running thought or theme is, realize the complete opposite is waiting to be acknowledged and created by you.

If this seems counter-intuitive, think about it this way: the doubts are training you to believe in yourself and to love yourself in whatever area by using the opposite message. For example, if you hear, "I can't make enough money in this business venture," that's a great test and a sign to strengthen your resolve until your goals are realized. Accept this "apparently negative truth" and look at this doubt as a reminder that you have forgotten to truly believe in yourself. It's time to pump up your thoughts and your heart's yearnings and goals by engaging active faith and feeling as if your goal is already realized.

As you understand this concept of befriending the doubts, your life will change. Your job is to monitor each and every thought, and instead of swimming in the fears as they surface, interrogate them and question their underlying messages. You must learn to believe in yourself – especially when the doubts are strong and when there is no sign that your dream will become a reality. These intense feelings are telling you that something great is about to happen if you neutralize the doubt. Hang in there, keep working, and keep pumping up your excitement. Actually, doubts are connected to an internal program that lives in each one of us. As odd as this may seem, the doubts are proof that Source / God is alive within you, desiring for you to choose happiness and recognize that every doubt is inviting you to connect with the Divine.

On the subject of Divine, many folks have found that calling God forth seems too big, and they are not able to make an emotional connection. Yet, a profound shift of feeling the Divine occurs when using the names Mom / Dad God in their affirmations / anchors. Many have commented that as parents they desire to see their children happy. So along with the idea that we have Earthly parents, we also have celestial parents, hence Mom and Dad God, who also strongly desire to see us (their children) happy. By mindfully turning our doubts around, it's like receiving a comforting memo to connect with the Divine.

If using the name God works for you, then by all means continue.

So repeat this out loud:

Expect to be challenged!

Expect to be challenged!

Expect to be challenged!

Get this; understand this. Learn to have fun with your doubts because each doubt contains great clues for you and your success. Look forward to the doubts as they are a constant reminder to course-correct and expand your Divine power.

If your doubts awaken you in the middle of the night, remind yourself to imagine and feel as though your goal has been realized. Never EVER forget what you are striving to achieve. Without a goal, you are aimless – a boat without a rudder – so try to be constantly aware of every thought. Your doubts will relentlessly make sure that you stand true while achieving your "seemingly impossible dreams."

Recognize, Renew, and Appreciate Your Choices

The doubts are asking, "Are you remembering to pump in the thought of joy and to nourish a sense of love for yourself with every breath you take?"

Remember, you have chosen happiness, so practice strengthening your conviction. Happiness is not hard to manufacture. It is simply new. Renounce complacency. Inspire yourself to awaken. **No one else can fight for your life but you!** Keep lifting out of your sludge. Become anew.

*"Insanity is doing the same
thing over and over again
and expecting different results."*

– Albert Einstein

Review your *Declaration to Self* and resolve to transform! This system of working with your doubts is alchemy at its highest level, turning all sourness or acidity into sweetness and happiness. Some of you may drink alkaline water throughout the day because it is health giving. Similarly, we are sipping our thoughts 24 hours a day, and many of the thoughts that "we hear in our head," are acidic, negative, and doubting – until we direct them. They test our resolve in order to gain our attention; it's up to us to turn those doubts into something more positive. The doubts are our great friends, our "inner trainers" like in the film series, *Rocky*. Mickey (Rocky's trainer and manager) loves Rocky and was training him to believe in himself and to be his best. So, rise. Actualize your potential and become the champion you are destined to be.

So, from 1–10 (10 being the most), how much desire do you have to turn your doubts inside out and realize your full potential? From 1–10, how motivated are you to take the action to accomplish this task? Your responses will tell you the level of your resolve. What would you do if you knew you couldn't fail?

Clearing the Slate: "Off-gassing"

When you stop "biting" into the doubts and stop making hurtful judgments towards yourself and

71

others, you may experience something we refer to as "off-gassing." This means that you are purging the judgments from your mind. You may feel worse as the old judgments are purged, so try saying, **"Clear the mechanism,"** **"no story,"** or, **"you are not real"** **as these intense sensations clear through your body.**

Don't attach yourself to or label the experience. Consider this as a new moment and let the old one go. See that these experiences were trainers for you to rise up and become the grandest self possible.

Consider transforming quickly – one moment at a time – not just one day at a time. If you are part of a 12-Step Program, know that you can actually "complete and delete" *(Chapter 7)* and be free of whatever lifelong story or pattern that haunts you by truly letting go of the old and stepping into the new.

Snuggle Up to Your Doubts

It's important to understand that doubts are present in your life to help you end the challenging stories – your war stories – forever. You may be a war veteran, or you might be struggling with alcohol, overeating, gambling, or coping with abuse as a child. We would never deny the terrible feelings associated with going through such horrendous experiences, yet, friends, don't stop there. Recognize that doubts are your friends, assisting to raise you up and help you move beyond the trauma, so you can emerge healthier, happier, and with a deeper more intimate connection with your partner and the Divine.

When you can begin to identify the resistances or doubts as signs that part of you is beckoning to be grander, please say, "Hi, my trainers." Instead of running from the voice that says that it's too scary, snuggle into it. When we fight with ourselves, we're like dogs safeguarding a play toy with clenched teeth, refusing to let go even as the toy is raised, carrying the dog into the air with it. It's time to let go of the unsatisfying clench. Move right into the resistance because more brilliance is waiting. It's safe to accept the doubts, fears, and insecurities and to embrace them. Give them a big metaphorical hug and say, "Thanks for awakening me." This ends the "Tug of War."

Wendy's Personal Story About Overcoming Overeating

A number of years ago, I struggled with my weight and controlling my food intake. I was working through emotional issues as well at the time. I joined a 12-Step Program – Overeating Anonymous – and diligently worked the steps with the help of a wonderful sponsor.

The funny thing was that during these months at OA I had more food binges than I ever experienced! I noticed that the more I denied myself the foods I was craving, the more I pigged out. I was determined to figure this issue out! I left OA and shortly after received a life-changing book, Overcoming Overeating, by Jane R. Hirschmann and Carol H. Munter, from a dear friend.

I closely followed this book's advice, which was to befriend all of my fears about food. The author suggested going to the supermarket and filling up the shopping cart with all the foods I couldn't seem to control – chunky peanut butter, ice cream, cookies, cake, etc. I was so embarrassed and ashamed as I displayed all of my "bad foods" at the check-out counter. I allowed myself to pig out for days, as the book suggested I eat until I no longer wanted to anymore.

How scary to be that out of control and watching my weight soar! But I kept allowing myself to be out of control. After a couple of weeks I came into an amazing balance and peace with myself. By allowing myself to have fun with food, I naturally stopped binging.

We know from our own experience that the more we allow ourselves to be happy that we will no longer have addictions to suffering, rather, we will develop addictions to happiness. The key is in the allowing and the accepting.

Try to remember what doubt was surfacing when you started to overeat, drink too much, or use drugs, etc. Is it possible that instead of being addicted to food, sex, drugs, etc., we are just not used to living in unconditional happiness?

The love you are seeking has always been inside of you. By clearing out the doubts, the sheaths of cloudy, heavy, numb feelings around your emotional heart will melt away and you will feel a joy and love in your body at unprecedented levels. That's juicy!

As electrical current runs though our bodies consider the idea that we magnetize our thoughts. Picture a magnet. Put a few pieces of paper at the end of the magnet. Then take another magnet and place it on the other side of the paper. Do the two magnets join together? No. Why? The paper, which represents our doubts, fears, judgments, etc., keeps the two magnets from attaching to each other.

Now, by using the *Turn Your Doubts Inside Out* technique (to be described at the end of this chapter), you will quickly be able to transform your doubts and fears. By doing this, you'll be figuratively removing the paper sheaths, and the magnets come together.

The clearer we are, the quicker we are able to manifest our desires.

Science has shown that it can take up to thirty days of consistent affirmations to transform a deeply rooted negative thought / pattern in our brain's neural network. So, be patient yet consistent and have compassion for yourself as you evolve into a more beautiful person while manifesting your desires. As you transform, you are doing your part in a Revolution of Love that is awakening on our planet. This new, joyous you and juicy relationship will have a profound impact on Earth. We can only imagine how proud and pleased Mother Earth is for you as you become mindful of ending your war of negativity. May this spread, so inappropriate behavior like bullying, physical abuse, shootings, and war cease.

Call to Action

Write out your doubts and their underlying messages. For example:

Doubt #1 – <u>What does the doubt say?</u> *My dream of paying off all my debt is impossible, and I'm in the clouds even wishing for this dream to come true. After all, I'm struggling to make my monthly payments, never mind clearing my debt.*

<u>What's the doubt's real purpose for showing up?</u> *To remind me that my dream of financial success is on its way. I'm choosing to feel that my desires to clear all financial debt are already realized, and I choose to keep pumping this goal in my awareness all day long.*

<u>Any action I need to take?</u> *To remember to focus on the gratitude of the finances that I do have now and the way that I have set out a plan to make my dreams a reality. Also, I'm going to empower all people to realize their financial dreams as well.*

DOUBT #1 - What does the doubt say?

_____

_____

_____

_____

What is the doubt's real purpose for showing up? Turn it inside out.

_____

_____

_____

_____

Any action I need to take?

_____

_____

_____

_____

DOUBT #2 - What does the doubt say?

_____

_____

_____

_____

What is the doubt's real purpose for showing up? Turn it inside out.

_____

_____

_____

_____

Any action I need to take?

_____

_____

_____

_____

"Anchor" – The Secret Word That Brings Instant Joy

Wouldn't it be wonderful to have a key phrase or word that could instantly shift your state of being from sad to glad? The secret is to engage a powerful mood shifter that we call an "anchor" which activates active faith.

- "Anchors" are strengthening thoughts or affirmations you repeat continually to yourself, like a mantra.

- These thoughts or ideas make you exuberantly happy, make your heart smile, and inspire you to keep rising out of sleepiness, despair, and any and all fears.

- Any time a doubt comes in that's a sign that you need to remember to put your "anchors" in.

- If you find that an "anchor" is no longer working for you, that's an indicator that you are climbing up your mountain of joy. Step up your conviction to rise through the density of intensity. An exciting new level of manifestation is being birthed and you will feel this!

- Keep pumping yourself up with <u>new</u> inspiring exalting "anchors."

Here are some possible "anchors:"

- I choose to be happy now.

- I choose to be happy so that my celestial Mom and Dad will chuckle knowing that one of their kids is happy.

- I choose to emanate exuberance into my environment – my partner, family, co-workers, and team are happy when I'm happy, and they value my joyous presence in their lives now.

- I now choose to access money from my unlimited account in "The Bank of the Divine" for my financial success and to benefit myself and others. Happy, thank you, more please.

- Everywhere I go, I now choose to bring a huge wave of joy. (This is a great one for performers, those in business, moms and dads, teachers, or anyone in a service-oriented profession).

- I choose to make my joyful smile infectious now.

- I now choose to plant vibrant cocoons of happiness ahead of me in every room, office, plane, store, etc. which I walk into.

- I choose to send forth a cocoon emanating happiness to permeate a city, house, country, and the Earth now. I now choose to access this power for the good of all.

- Every second, I choose to be preparing for a ball now.

- My partner and I choose to live in a constant honeymoon glow now.

- I now choose to be tickled pink to be me.

- Every second, I now choose to feel the joy of Christmas morning.

"I've wrestled with reality, doctor, for 40 years now, and I finally overcame it!"

– Jimmy Stewart as "Elwood Dowd"
in the movie, *Harvey*

You may notice a pattern of repetition with the words "I choose" and "now." Saying "I choose" is declaring your "vote" or your desire, and saying "now" engages and puts your anchor into action of active faith immediately. Your subconscious mind likes to be given a "job" and will now work continuously to manifest your wishes.

Now it's time to discover what your particular "anchors" are and how to use them to transform your life. You'll be excited about using your "anchors" because when you stop pumping in the thoughts and desires you want, the doubts get engaged to remind you to do so. They come knocking at the door saying, "Hey, wake up!"

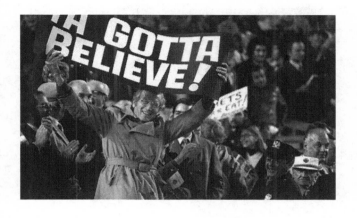

My "anchors" are:

_____

_____

_____

_____

_____

_____

_____

_____

_____

_____

_____

_____

_____

_____

_____

How often do you deal with your doubts? Daily, multiple times during a day, weekly?

The World on Your Shoulders

Have your doubts ever affected your intimate relationships or been the cause of a fight or a break up? How often are you dueling with your doubts to rid them from your life? Do you find that sometimes the doubts go away, but they always seem to pop back up, especially when you get excited and inspired about doing something new? By not having a guaranteed system to transform fears, doubts, and insecurities quickly, you probably feel the heavy weight of the world on your shoulders.

Throughout your life, how many times have you listened to the DOUBT and believed it and found yourself feeling heavy or depressed? Once, a few times, constantly? Has it ever slowed or even sabotaged your desires? If you took an inventory of the time you spent dealing with your doubts (journaling, therapy, talking with friends, etc.), would it amount to a lot of time? What would it feel like if you drastically reduced the time you spent dealing with your doubts and experienced more joyous moments instead?

The Well of Despair

How many times have you neutralized the out of control, spiraling heavy feelings of doubt, then put the opposite thought in your head and felt renewed in five minutes or less? For example, "I choose to feel beautiful now," "I choose to be successful with my work now," "I choose to please my partner now," or, "I choose to know I am a loving parent now."

Are You Ready to End the War?

A negative thought occurs. It's a memo/messenger trying to get your attention. Thoughts happen so quickly that you don't realize you have aligned with them and bitten into the "poisoned apple." The sourness comes into you, and you start to feel a blackened energy in your body. Uncomfortable feelings arise in the belly, neck, shoulders, back, jaw, etc. Do you like the way it feels when you have bitten into the doubt? It's YOUR choice not to bite into this poison. Be aware that the feelings ONLY start when you have bitten into the DOUBT.

Doubts Harm Artists, Athletes, and Businesses

You probably have heard stories of how the doubts in singers, songwriters, actors, dancers etc. have negatively impacted their craft and ability to enjoy their life. Many performers have been known to throw up due to nerves before a show. Athletes have lost their focus when doubts arise, and they have affected their ability to be successful, especially in a huge event. Business people lose opportunities and money due to their doubts.

Cary loves the game of golf and studies how the mental approach plays a role in a golfer's success. You can literally watch the positive or negative effect of how a player is dealing with their "inner game." One of the best men to ever play the game, Bobby Jones, has been often quoted saying, "Competitive golf is played mainly on a five-and-a-half-inch course, the space between your ears."

Often, a tournament is won not by the difference in the physical talent in the field, but by a player's ability to transform doubts while playing. As more golfers learn to get excited, realizing that the doubts are training and preparing them for a transformative breakthrough, they will start to feel more confident in their abilities and experience more success. From weekend warriors to touring professionals, golfers have sought out Cary's coaching on how to champion their inner game to success.

Shocking Body-Image News:

97% of Women Will Be Cruel to Their Bodies Today

~ Shaun Dreisbach, Glamour Magazine
reprinted with permission
Complete article is included in Appendix G

Scary but true: exclusive glamour survey, young women recorded an average of 13 brutal thoughts about their bodies each day. We say: Enough!

Read these words: "You are a fat, worthless pig." "You're too thin. No man is ever going to want you." "Ugly. Big. Gross." Horrifying comments on some awful website? The rant of an abusive, controlling boyfriend? No; shockingly, these are the actual words young women are saying to themselves on any typical day.

For some, such thoughts are fleeting, but for others, this dialogue plays on a constant, punishing loop, according to a new exclusive *Glamour* survey of more than 300 women of all sizes.

Our research found that, on average, women have 13 negative body thoughts daily—nearly one for every waking hour. And a disturbing number of women confess to having 35, 50 or even 100 hateful thoughts about their own shapes each day.

Would you like to transform your doubts and experience more pleasure and success personally and professionally? Would you like to never again have to spend lots of time dueling with your doubts? If so, let's proceed to the 5-step system of Turning Your Doubts Inside Out Forever!

TURN YOUR DOUBTS INSIDE OUT™

This is our 5-step system to turn your doubts and fears around forever.

1. Get Excited – Doubts are your friends not your enemies.

2. Accept the Doubt – Say, "It's a truth, not the only truth." a few times out loud or silently.

3. Stop biting into negative thoughts, which create a heaviness in your body.

4. Repeat, "Feelings are my friends," over and over like a mantra. Emphasize a different word each time: "*Feelings* are my friends," "Feelings *are* my friends," etc. until the heaviness dissipates to a four or less on a scale from 1–10, and you begin to feel yourself return to a calm state.

5. Now, and only now, say the opposite. It may feel forced or mechanical at first as the new neural net in your brain is being created. Say "I choose to feel beautiful now," "I choose to be financially successful now," "I choose to effortlessly reach my goals now," "I choose to please my partner intimately now," etc.

Take a photo with your phone of the 5 steps so you can access them at all times. This will be very helpful when a strong doubt comes, and you are emotionally overwhelmed. All you'll need to do is pull up the photo and follow the steps.

Now you know you have a choice, a roadmap, to remind you that there's a new glorious place to move towards, bringing you to more and more radiant happiness. That's exciting! Turn your doubt inside out, and give yourself the gift of unconditional love. As you keep working with yourself 24 hours a day, pumping in effervescent happiness, we guarantee 100 percent that you will feel changes in your body. It's amazing, truly amazing!

The Stronger Your Doubts, the Stronger Your Gifts, Talent, and Purpose

Doubts arise to get your attention, reminding you to strengthen your connection / relationship with the Divine. Whatever the doubt says, the **exact** opposite is the truth, such as:

"I'm not beautiful." / "I'm too fat." = "I AM voluptuously beautiful."

"I'll never make enough money." = Success is awaiting you.

When you utilize the Turn Your Doubts Inside Out System, you'll never feel alone / lonely / cutoff EVER again! You will feel more joy, juiciness, and success. And your connection with Source will grow stronger than ever before!

Ever Felt Zapped?

Have you ever been doing something creative like writing a song or a book, painting, or inventing when all of a sudden you felt extremely tired? So tired that you didn't even have the energy to walk to your bed? You just instantly fell asleep wherever you were?

If this ever happens to you, realize that this is the Divine desiring for you to connect with its presence. You're probably asking, "Okay, but what do I do?" Immediately connect with Source. Say, "God," or "Mom/Dad God, I choose to have you assist me with my creation. Thank you for your presence and love in my life. Please send more now. Happy, thank you, more please."

After you say the "anchor," the tiredness will magically go away, and you won't need to sleep. Very profound! Happy creation making.

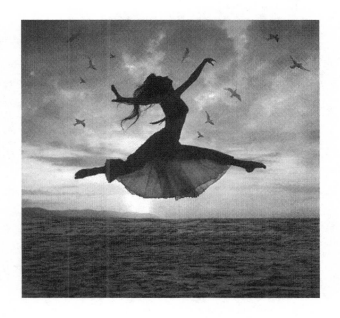

CHAPTER SUMMARY POINTS

*"To be fully seen by somebody,
then, and beloved anyhow –
this is a human offering that
can border on miraculous."*

~ Elizabeth Gilbert

• Begin to recognize your doubts. Your job is
  to monitor each and every thought, and instead
  of swimming in the fears as they surface,

interrogate them and understand
their underlying messages.

- Stop the doubt in its tracks. Accept what it says
with a smile on your face and start pumping in
the opposite.

- When you stop pumping in your dream /
"anchor," that's when the doubts come
knocking at the door saying, "Hey,
wake up!"

- As we fill ourselves with sunshine and
activate active faith, we will find our
addictions naturally drop away, and we
can enjoy all things with sincere gratitude
and balance. These tools will give you the
strength to move beyond the labels of a
particular addiction forever. Give thanks
to the Creator numerous times daily by
saying "happy, thank you, more please,
Divine Creator".

- If you are going to doubt something,
doubt your limits.

- 90 day journey: Discontinue "biting" into
your doubts and reacting negatively to each
other. Past hurts in the relationship start to
clear, preparing you to "complete and delete"
the past issues.

- For inspiration in dealing with doubts,
  watch the films *Brother Sun, Sister Moon;
  A Beautiful Mind; Seven Days In Utopia;
  and The Sunshine Makers (cartoon).*

Click the link below to access tools and tips
on championing the inner game of golf at
Raise The Cup.

The War Is Over!

Today, I declare the war is over.
The war is complete.
I have found the enemy – it is me.
I have found my greatest friend – it is me.

Today, I declare the war of doubt is over.
Doubt is one of my best friends, not my enemy.

Doubt is one of my greatest trainers of loving self.
Doubt has not come to take me down the well of emotional abyss.

Doubt has come to test my desire,
to see how strong I believe in what I say or dream.
The storm of Doubt has come.
Its deepest desire is to help me make sure I stand by my heart's yearnings.

The storm of Doubt desires strongly that I succeed,
yet it must present turbulence to me,
the exact opposite of what it desires for me.

The storm of Doubt is my sparing partner –
the stronger and closer I get to realizing my dreams,
the stronger the storm gets.
It must keep intensifying, staying one step ahead.

The storms may shorten, yet their blows will be more intense.
Doubt is one of my greatest trainers of accepting all of me.

Whenever a doubt arises,
I remember it has come to remind me to love myself.
Doubt is not my enemy; it is one of my best friends.

Chapter 4

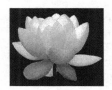

Secret 3a – Make a Huge Impact on Your Mate Without Saying a Word

"I believe that everything happens for a reason. People change so that you can learn to let go, things go wrong so that you appreciate them when they're right, you believe lies so you eventually learn to trust no one but yourself, and sometimes good things fall apart so better things can fall together."

~ Marilyn Monroe

Before proceeding further, let's address a frequently asked question: What do you do if one partner wants to grow and the other is resistant? If your partner feels that everything is fine in the relationship, or does not want to talk about the questions in chapter one, or is not interested in hearing about your concerns or your yearnings to grow, take note. Perhaps your partner feels uneasy about opening up about his or her emotions and, therefore, feels a bit resistant about even hearing you bring the subject up.

A great solution is to **write a letter** from your heart. Writing down your thoughts can help you clearly express your ideas without the other's influence. Be honest and explain things that matter to you, things about yourself and your partner, and about what you truthfully see happening between the two of you.

Write about what's happened in your relationship with the hope and intent that the letter will really touch your partner. Do not blame him or her for your feelings. Focus on the <u>behavior</u> that challenges you, not on the person.

You may well need to write with a very strong tone to shake up the situation in order to convince your partner how much he or she means to you. This kind of intensity is often what it takes to crack the shell of repetitive patterns. Dare to reveal your honest feelings.

If your partner is still not willing to explore these areas with you, consider opening up to something new in your life. Maybe the relationship needs to go in a new direction, perhaps one that involves no longer being together. Do everything you can to revive your relationship. Yet, if there are no signs of positive movement and desire to improve, be prepared to let it all go. Life is too precious to be with someone who <u>chooses</u> not to better himself / herself and the relationship.

The relationship of your dreams is awaiting you; it just might not be with your present partner. Here's something to consider, and it may reveal an answer that you're not ready to hear. Ask yourself: "What am I getting from the relationship, if I'm not able to communicate and be intimate and juicy with my partner?" This is a soul-searching time.

You must decide what is important to you. This is a time to stretch beyond your comfort zone with the intent of being happier. Being sublimely happy. You know when you feel stuck and unhappy or when you feel inspired. Trust your gut feelings. Support is always available if you really want to grow and transform. Again, ask yourself: "Do I want to grow and renew this relationship, and can I do this with my partner?"

If you are considering ending your relationship, begin by exploring all other possible options to turn over a new leaf together. Perhaps a separation will help by giving you time to figure yourselves out. Make a conscious decision to make divorce the very last option because no matter who you choose to be with next, you will most likely face your same concerns again if they are still a part of you.

Of course, there is nothing wrong with divorce and starting again, though it is often very tough and emotionally and financially disruptive. If there are children involved, consider having a discussion with them about how they feel about this change.

It's important to tackle these obstacles now instead of repeating the same patterns in your next relationship. Snuggle up to the obstacles – don't run from them – because their job is to train you to grow, and these challenges will find a way to show up in your next relationship. Obstacles are your friends, not your enemies; they help you to grow and to become stronger.

Just know that any partnership will require work, commitment, and an understanding of how to own your patterns without blaming the other person. Think about how you initially felt about each other. Have you grown? If you are married, are you being true to your wedding vows?

Anyone who has participated with someone else in a sport such as mountain climbing learns that everyone must carry their own weight and battle for their lives. Think of your relationship in a similar way. You are connected to each other by an imaginary rope. Each person takes turns leading the way, sometimes pulling the weight for the other person as he or she gathers strength, so that, eventually, you both walk side by side.

A partnership is a brilliant way to help each other make positive changes. Why not suggest to your partner that you both read this book together?

The Silent Divorce

Now here's a tough question we would like you to reflect on. Are you living a <u>silent</u> divorce? Have you structured your lives to avoid intimacy? Do you both live very separate busy lives? You may unknowingly be avoiding difficult unresolved issues, but the feelings will eventually emerge in unhealthy patterns. It is never too late to change!

Do you hear yourself saying any of the following when describing your marriage to others: "All is great; all is wonderful; it's all good. We never have any disagreements or problems between us." Since most people have said these things about their own marriages in the past, they tend to believe that you're not being truthful. Perhaps you need coaxing to admit your fears, insecurities, and challenges.

Think about something for a minute: Did any of us ever get a "how-to" guide in high school, college, or beyond explaining ways to have an incredible relationship? The majority of us can probably benefit from enhanced intimate relationship skills, especially if we keep finding ourselves putting out fires in our relationships.

You may have more experience in the area of communication than your partner. Consider easing him or her into exploring and opening up. Encourage your partner to take even the smallest steps. Help him or her see that the purpose of opening up is to embrace greater and greater levels of happiness.

After all, most of us have invested years and years in habitual negative patterns, and we are accustomed to living with fear and unhappiness. Step by step, we can choose to develop new positive ways of thinking and relating to each other and ourselves. Over time, these new ways will become automatic. A happy, fulfilling partnership is slowly crafted through desire and dedication and is available to all who yearn to live in sublime sweetness.

Do you want to stay in dull, repetitious, unfulfilling, unjuicy lives, or are you willing to risk opening up to something new? Are you tired of your unhappy states of being? We are only as happy as our level of self acceptance, which is fueled by the passionate desire to actualize our dreams.

The difference between accepting things as they are and wishing they were different is the tiny distance between heaven and hell. Life is just waiting for us to believe in ourselves. We can craft a spectacular life by developing our unique gifts. So, what will you choose?

The following is a letter that Cary wrote to Wendy at 3 a.m. during a night when he couldn't sleep at a very difficult turning point in their married life.

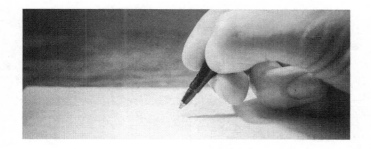

Declaration to Life

My Dear Wendy,

I've been afraid, afraid for years, of confronting you with the contents of this letter. I know this is going to sound crazy. I truly felt you would be so angered by what I am about to say that you would literally bite my head off, chew on it, and spit it out in disgust. But now I don't care if you or anyone else comes to kill me because I already feel dead. We are dead; what do I have to lose? So here goes.

This moment seems to have spun and spun and spun again. What moment you ask? The moment of darting hateful, crushing, biting energies at each other. Aren't you sick of this? The feelings are horrendous. We have both been harsh to each other, even vile.

What I am wanting most from you is HONESTY. A simple touch of care, a smile. A "hey friend/lover; how are you?" And from the tone of your voice I feel your love.

What's happened to our romance? Our intimacy has dried up. Where did your vibrant enthusiasm and lust for life go? I know I am messed up, too, yet neither of us can get anywhere new until you, my lady, look into your heart and transform.

I want us to flourish as happy, romantic lovers. This may sound crude, but my heart lies in my hard-on. When we are not engaged sexually, something in me turns off, and I feel like I'm dying. I am not talking just hot wild sex here. I'm talking from a place of our sweet, loving connection.

Right now, you're probably looking to defend yourself. Don't. Don't even try. LISTEN. Hear with an open heart, a feeling heart. I am your lover. I desire so much to care and nurture you, to help pull out the metaphorical shards of broken glass embedded in your heart. I feel you so deeply. What's locked up in you is also locked up in me, and we can't get anywhere until you turn the key.

Your tormented heart has been with you for eons. Certainly long before you met me. I want to be with you, to help pull the shards from your heart, and with each one released, I want to watch the blood of life return. I don't care if I'm injured in the process. All I want is to watch your passionate, kind heart reawaken.

This is a desperate hour. Your life is at stake. Not just yours, mine as well. We are linked together,

*whether we like it or not. I will either die or leave you.
And as challenging, painful, and scary as it would be
for me to leave you, I will. I must, as I won't let myself
for one more second die of a broken heart.*

*I know somehow, we are meant for greatness
together. Great love. Great friendship. I wonder if I
could ever find another woman in this tired old world
that I'd feel the same way about. Yet, I also wonder if
there is more waiting for me. Can there be a woman
out there in the world that would embrace me and
take me to places in my heart of desires that would
surpass what you could?*

*I need your loving support. If I have a business
idea, truly support me instead of saying, "I don't like
the idea, so don't do it," or "go ahead, but I'm not
really behind it." I know I am not perfect. I'm not
happy with how I've treated you at times either. I need
to make changes, too. I will be more honest with you
when you do or say things that push my buttons. I'll
stop lashing out. We'll discover where we went off
course, where we were hurt by a jealous thought, and
where fear or doubt hindered our happiness.*

*My love, what do you want? Do you want to
change, or are you afraid to break from convention?
What is your choice? Listen to your heart not your
head. Are you going to throw out the truest love you
have ever known because you are afraid? Afraid that
you aren't perfect?*

We can figure out how not to be run by these thoughts anymore, how to not "bite" into the poisoned apple of hatred that spirals us down a well of despair. We can rediscover our hearts and that all-encompassing love we have for each other. And we can get back to telling each other how much we care for one another. This alone will alter the feeling in our home.

If your answer is "Yes! Let's fix this," then what do you say about figuring it out like two little kids making sand castles? We'll choose to stop blaming our feelings on each other. We'll stop yelling at each other.

Will you choose to create an amazing life with me and work through our challenges together or not? Now, right now, you need to make a choice. What will it be? Make your choice and don't look back.

Cary

Wendy responded to the letter:

Yes. Yes. A million times, yes. I am profoundly sorry; I didn't realize how rigid and stuck I've become, how afraid I've been to be happy, how self-absorbed I've become. I've been so afraid to love for fear of losing. Why bother because I will then have to eventually suffer and say goodbye. So, I've stayed stuck in my fear.

I am making a declaration right now, with you as my witness, to change. I will not be the woman I was ever again. I will open up and let go of the old crappy stories. I call forth strength to transform. I vow to be a lover to myself and to you.

Deeply touched, we embraced and shared gut-wrenching cries, kissing deeply as lovers, wet with tears. Giggling, we set off hand in hand to forge a new adventure together.

Well, there you have it. This is our true story. Can you relate? Do you have a similar story? So many of us, as men and women, are separated from each other, whether we are living together or apart. The divorce rate is getting out of hand.

The good news is that we, ourselves, didn't get a divorce, even though there were many moments when we both wanted to! We learned how to work out the problems in our relationship, and now you are also figuring out your situation step by step with this groundbreaking system.

Consider writing a letter to get everything down on paper. It will crystallize where you and your partner stand in your relationship. You will quickly see how much your partner really wants to grow, transform, renew, and work together with you. It's time to get clear!

Call to Action
A Letter to My Partner

Before writing your letter, think about the following guidelines:

From 1–10, how happy are you in your present partnership? _____

What specifically do you want to see change in order for the relationship to move forward? i.e. What behavior would I like to see my partner transform?

_____

_____

_____

What behavior will I transform myself?

_____

_____

_____

Are you willing to put your relationship on the line by expressing your desires?

_____

_____

_____

What if your partner does not want to grow and transform? Will you stay true to your words?

_____

_____

_____

What kind of support do you need to make lasting change?

_____

_____

_____

_____

_____

_____

_____

_____

_____

Now, on the following page, write your partner a letter from your heart.

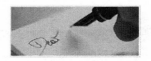

A Letter to My Partner

_____

_____

_____

_____

_____

_____

_____

_____

_____

_____

_____

_____

_____

_____

_____

_____

_____

_____

_____

CHAPTER SUMMARY POINTS

"Love doesn't make the world go round.
Love is what makes the ride worthwhile."

~ Franklin P. Jones

- Consider writing a letter to your partner, perhaps with a very strong yet loving tone, to get a clear understanding about where your relationship is heading and how you want to see it change.

- Snuggle up to the obstacles; don't run from them.

- Try easing your partner into exploring and opening up. Encourage him or her to take even small steps.

- A happy, fulfilling partnership is crafted over time through desire and dedication and is available to all who yearn to live in sublime sweetness.

- Resolve to move beyond dull, repetitious, unfulfilling, unjuicy patterns. Risk opening up to something new.

- Watch the films *Jerry Maguire* and *It's a Wonderful Life.*

- 90 day journey: Continue using and
  strengthening the foundational tools from
  the first 30 days. Master "the doubts" system.
  Feel a renewed sense of love and vitality in
  your relationship. Deepen your emotional and
  physical intimacy and have fun date nights.

Chapter 5

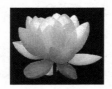

Secret 3b – The Love Agreement

"Marriage is a mosaic you build with your spouse. Millions of tiny moments that create your love story."

~ Jennifer Smith

The Contract

Once you have decided that you both want to grow and transform, we highly recommended that you make an official declaration to one another by signing and dating the following contract. For singles, sign the **Declaration to Self**, and for couples, please sign **The Love Agreement for Couples.**

There is great power in firmly committing to this process of deepening your level of happiness with each other and life itself. By putting your commitment in writing, you empower one another to make the choices necessary to improve and grow as partners.

These agreements are a reminder to hold each other to your heartfelt commitment, so that you don't go back to your old patterns. These contracts will keep you grounded and present. They are not a punishment, nor are they here to harm or hurt you. They simply recognize your commitment and help support you in your efforts to change and to build the new glorious partnership of your dreams.

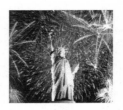

DECLARATION TO SELF

I agree to take full responsibility for all of my thoughts and actions and will not blame any outside circumstance for my unhappiness (i.e. how I look, the economy, the weather).

I agree to stop "biting" into the poisoned apple of fear, doubt, and worry now as I realize my choices affect everyone I come in contact with.

I agree to appropriately manage myself and handle any intense feelings that arise, knowing these feelings are a memo reminding me to pump up my happiness, deepen my connection with God / Divine, and create my dreams.

I choose to stay honest and keep eliminating my judgments about myself and others as I prepare for my future partnership.

I choose to create an exalted joyous life now and to fill myself up with effervescent happiness every second of the day.

Signature   Date

THE LOVE AGREEMENT FOR COUPLES

I agree to take full responsibility for all of my thoughts and actions and will not blame my partner or any outside circumstance for my unhappiness (i.e. how I look, the economy, the weather).

I agree to stop "biting" into the poisoned apple of fear, doubt, and worry as I realize my choices affect my partner, my family, and the world.

I agree to appropriately manage myself and handle any intense feelings that arise, knowing these feelings are a memo reminding me to pump up my happiness, deepen my connection with God / Divine, and create my dreams.

I choose to create an exalted joyous life with my partner now and to fill myself up every second of the day with effervescent happiness.

At all times, we commit to ensuring that each of us is upholding this contract. We each agree to shake one another out of any complacency, so that we can reach our greatest potential. We agree to regularly review and update this agreement.

_____

Signature   Date

_____

Signature   Date

Chapter 6

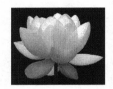

Secret 4 – Your Body Has Feelings, Too

"Love is of all passions the strongest, for it attacks simultaneously the head, the heart and the senses."

~ Lao Tzu

We will now address feelings and emotions and how to tell when you are creating them versus releasing them. Our physical bodies are vastly affected by our thoughts. For example, how do you feel inside your body when you are happy? How about when you are worried or critical of yourself or others?

Every thought is a subtle form of energy and gets recorded in the physical body. Worry and fear are some of the most intensified thought forms, and their energy is associated with uncomfortable feelings in the body, such as stress, headaches, stomach aches, backaches, the onset or worsening of a disease, or simply feeling emotionally dull or numb.

As you begin to let go of your own particular worry and fear pattern, you will often feel a physical/emotional release. We call this "unwinding," the sensation that occurs when you release fear from your body. Instead of immediately calling the doctor when you experience these sensations, just relax. Allow the time for the sensations to take their course of arising and releasing. The mind will often search for a reason why the body is reacting in such a way. For instance: "Could it be something I ate? Maybe I lifted something too heavy." Try to refrain from engaging these "stories." If you find yourself reacting in a story, simply stop, breathe, and visualize your body as healed.

Practice witnessing the sensations in your body. Dive right into the sensations without trying to stop the release. You may find yourself teary-eyed when these intense sensations or even memories are emerging. Again, allow the release! This is a great moment. You are clearing out your "hard drive," so to speak.

We have noticed that as we cleared out patterns of fear, worry, or doubt in our own bodies, many aches and pains came and went. Over time, we learned not to react to the sudden discomfort in our bodies, such as backaches or knee aches. Although we sometimes felt like a train had run over us, inside our hearts we celebrated because we knew that fear was clearing out and leaving us for good.

The Body Is Neutral

The body is a blank slate waiting to be directed. Repeat this concept over and over to yourself: "My body is neutral. My body is neutral. It responds 100 percent to the thoughts I am holding at any given moment." As you let go of fear, your body will respond accordingly.

You are beginning to see how extraordinarily powerful you are. Whatever you have been creating has been based on how you think and feel about yourself. You are the most powerful pharmacologist in the world. Your judgments have a huge impact on you and even on your children. Have you ever asked your child what kind of birthday cake he or she wants? Don't children usually get excited about their favorite flavor of cake with lots of frosting and some kind of fun design like a rocket or a mermaid? Rarely does a child say, "Mom, I'll have a bowl of kale with a candle in it." Children teach us to be in touch with the excitement and passion of the moment, to live perpetually in the Christmas-like spirit. What a great way to focus on our passionate creations, rather than the countless things we could be afraid of.

Do you ever remember playing outside as a child, maybe making a fort in the snow? Perhaps you had a runny nose, but you didn't even think about it because you were so enraptured with building that fort. Perhaps your mom saw your runny nose and made you come inside. Yes, moms are very attuned to their children's needs, but they must also be careful not to superimpose their fears onto their husbands and children.

Children intuitively understand that happiness is an exalted state of being. Try to learn from them and remember to keep pumping up the happiness factor. *Your greatest gift to your child or spouse is your choice to be happy.* And by making the decision to live in a state of happiness, the necessary solutions to any given situation will become very clear, very quickly.

Let's review the maps in the Appendix for a moment. Life shows up, and you may initially judge and react to it. For example, while looking in the mirror you may feel, "I'm not beautiful enough." We call that thought a doubt. What you do with that doubt will set your course of action in motion.

If you take that doubt at face value and "bite" into the poisoned apple, you are going to feel "squirts" of feelings throughout your body. Maybe these will be new sensations. Perhaps you never realized the effect that "biting" into this doubt had on your overall energy.

Once you recognize this, your feelings will show you where you are traveling. For example, perhaps you lost a lot of money in the stock market and are worried about what may happen in the future, so you spend all your time looking at the market on the computer, so obsessed that you can't rest. You may feel this literally in your stomach and might simply label it stress. Then, out of the blue, you learn you have an ulcer. Consider that you may have created that ulcer by believing in the fear or doubt that all your money was going to drain away. You "bit" into the fear that perhaps you'd be living in the poor house in a cardboard box under a bridge.

Now, let's look at this scenario from a different perspective. Life shows up, and the stock market plummets. Instead of reacting, take a moment and accept the state of affairs that you may end up in. You cannot control the ups and downs of the stock market, but you can control how you react to it.

This scenario beckons you to consciously grow and expand. Take a breath and accept the possibility that you could, indeed, end up living on the street without a clue as to where your money would come from. If you are willing to face and feel what you are most afraid of – i.e. becoming impoverished and homeless – then you won't need to create such scenarios. Why not have fun while imagining living on the street?

Instead of focusing on the fear of living on the street, use your imagination to create what you really desire. How about repeating to yourself, "Financial surprises are coming my way." By doing so, you move to the right side of the map – *The Wheel of Manufacturing Happiness*. *This lighthearted approach will help deflate the power of the fear and will help you let go of the tug of war inside you.*

You can be certain that the stronger the doubt, the greater the opportunity for financial abundance. The uncomfortable feelings function as a kind of checkpoint, a messenger, beckoning you to look deeply at your life and possibly the kind of work you are doing. Ask yourself, "Is this really what I want to be doing?"

Is My Present Work Aligned with My Dream and Purpose?

If you had $10 million in the bank (or enough money for you to live on), what kind of work would you be passionate about? Are you just focusing on survival or are you developing your own original, "authentic swing?" When you stop reacting to the fear of survival, you literally free yourself and begin to create something new.

Cary's Personal Story of Fear and Insight

For such a long time, I had been haunted by money and survival fears. Over the years, I worked through my fears of not having enough money, and at one point I chose to live very simply like a monk. Years later, after returning to society and working again, I surprisingly found this same fear crop up.

One day as I was walking through the supermarket, I felt a strangling constriction in my throat and was overwhelmed with a gut-wrenching fear over purchasing milk and cookies for myself and Wendy. At that moment, our monthly expenses exceeded our monthly income by a few thousand dollars, and we were uncertain of the future of our work.

The crazy thing was that at that exact moment **we had $23,000 in our checking account!**

Yet, I felt as if I didn't have the money to pay for these items. The fear was that the money was dwindling. I know that this paralyzing fear makes no sense. However, it was very real. The point of the realization was to turn these doubts inside out.

As I was walking down the cookie and cracker aisle, I silently asked myself, "What is going on here? Why am I feeling such intense pressure?" The response I heard inside my head was, "Your purpose, Cary, is to positively impact multitudes of people, and you will be well paid for that. You need to let go, 'clear' these money fears, and learn to be at ease at all times. You are right on track. You are reprogramming your beliefs and training yourself to believe in the original work that your heart so deeply wants to share with others."

Hearing these words, my heart burst open and, immediately, the fear and constriction evaporated. With that, I joyously bought the milk and cookies. I see now that although I wanted success, I was preparing for failure.

Later, I came home and talked to Wendy, admitting the fear that I would never be able to manifest my dream. I realized that the dream had always been waiting for me, but I first had to believe it. From this experience, I learned to let go of my focus on HOW my dreams were going to come true because I KNEW they were already on their way to coming true.

Wow! All this insight while in the grocery aisle! If you have such intense feelings, remind yourself not to "bite" into them. You are on your way to having your dreams. Try not to add to the fear. Relax. Allow the old fear program to disappear. When the feelings are very intense, you are close to changing a deep-seated pattern once and for all.

Oftentimes we are afraid to admit our fears, but, by admitting them, they will usually go away. If we hold in our fears because of shame, they will continue to pop up. So admit, admit. Admit what grabs you by the gonads, and you will find that the fear will go away.

As a reminder, if you are experiencing a doubt/fear pattern that you recognize is recycling, consider doing a "complete and delete" session (presented in the next chapter) with your partner or close friend.

Cary's situation is not out of the ordinary. When we lived in Santa Fe, New Mexico, a friend of ours shared a story with us about an acquaintance of his, a gentleman whose bank account dwindled to $1 million dollars, and he literally freaked out and didn't know how he was going to survive. He wrapped himself so tightly in this fearful story that he had to be put into a straitjacket and admitted to a mental institute.

So, what fears are you afraid to admit? How are you wrapping yourself in a straitjacket? Remember to lighten up and let go of the fear that is keeping you from believing in the fulfillment of your dreams.

"Your ships come in over a don't care sea."

– Florence Scovel Shinn

Let's go back for a moment and talk about the feelings in the body. When you look in the mirror and don't like what you see, you experience feelings in your body. You then begin to douse life, drain your energy, create unhappiness, and spin in the left wheel of the *Map of Choice*. If this happens, ask yourself how happy you are at that exact moment. What's so sexy about scrutinizing yourself with a furrowed brow?

When we fight with ourselves, our body starts reflecting our thoughts. Science has proven that the cells in our body take direct orders from our thoughts and have no sense of humor. The cells take every thought literally and are the biggest gossipers in the world, spreading your message to millions and millions of cells throughout your body. So choose your thoughts wisely and be very watchful of your fears because you will create what you think and feel most. The good news here is that your body will respond and change quickly in a positive way when you turn your doubts inside out and pump in the thoughts of what you want to create. (Note: For some interesting insight about health and marriage, see Tara Parker-Pope's *New York Times* article, "Is Marriage Good for Your Health?" in Appendix F.)

Inside Versus Outside – Doubts and Physical Appearance

A number of years ago, when Cary started to reveal his doubts, I was amazed at how much insecurity was running through him. Cary hid his fear quite well, whereas I tended to wear my insecurities on my sleeve. At that time, because I was more self-absorbed, I was not as able to perceive where he was at.

But now, because I have climbed out of my self-created ditch of misery, I can tell if he has "bitten" into a fear thought. I can sense it in his overall energy, as well as see worry in his face or eyes. The idea here is that the more honest and clear we become, the more we will be able to sense the present state of mind of another person. This is an important area to work on to keep the relationship growing and vibrant.

We may present ourselves to others positively on the outside, and yet inside there may be considerable turmoil going on behind the scenes – in the form of doubts, fears, and insecurities – and we may not even realize it.

Can you sense at any given moment what state of mind your partner or children are in? Make a commitment to monitor one another. There is no room for hiding out in your separate lonely corners. Make sure each family member is clearing his or her space and pumping themselves up with majestic thoughts. What we're talking about is a commitment to excellence, and there are amazing benefits, which come from caring at such a deep level.

Even though you may be a woman who is very physically appealing, if you are dealing with self-doubt and are consumed by always looking in the mirror and wanting to look perfect, then you may be projecting a degree of sourness in your energetic field. When we meet up with someone, we first see their physical appearance, yet we feel their energy even more so.

So many beautiful actresses and models on the magazine covers we see may look appealing. However, we may also sense an emptiness in those women, as many struggle internally with choosing to love themselves and appreciate their beauty. Some are constantly comparing themselves to other women. Have you ever thought that you are not as beautiful as your friends? How did that feel? Heavy, empty, or like an ominous dark cloud?

Imagine the doubts that go through such a person's mind as she looks in the mirror. She is continually fighting with the doubts she hears in her head, trying to appease these "biting" thoughts by constantly primping, exercising, and even resorting to surgical procedures to look more beautiful.

All she really wants is to <u>feel</u> beautiful, and the doubt is just trying to get her attention in order to remind her to love her own essence, her sweetness. All women carry this sweetness, regardless of how they may look. All girls and women are beautiful princesses, and there is genuine beauty within each of them just simply trying to bloom. It is the same for men. All boys and men are princes waiting to claim their gifts of regal glory.

Why Not Allow the Heart to Blossom?

Look at the Native American women elders who live in the southwest of the United States and who have spent a lot of time outside in the elements. Oftentimes, their faces reflect the effects of the desert. Physically, these women may not be as appealing as the cover girls. However, oftentimes, there is a sense of childlike innocence that shines through their weathered faces. You can feel a genuine sweetness radiating through their whole being.

You may be skeptical about this, especially if you're a man, and you may think this beauty issue is no big deal. But gentlemen, in all due respect for you and the women in your lives, consider having a conversation with them about how they feel about themselves and their looks.

If your intimacy with your lady has been disappointing, you may be surprised to find out that her lack of intimate desires has a lot less to do with you and a lot more to do with her judgments about her own body. She may be "biting" into the judgment that she is not beautiful, which will sour her desire to be juicy with you. So many marriages end in divorce because the intimacy wanes, and the man loses interest and seeks pleasure elsewhere. Having the conversation about the subject of looks and beauty is vital.

The exciting thing we're talking about here is being able to have it all – the physical beauty and the internal beauty. So sweet, so striking. Now that's a juicy, sexy, WOW! This is about falling in love with yourself, becoming your own lover. Once you do this, when you come together with your partner, you will be whole and overflowing, truly juicy like a ripe mango or fragrant like a sweet rose or gardenia.

As we clear out our baggage, we emanate an unworldly beauty anchored in love. This occurs when we deepen our partnership with the celestial realm: Divine Spirit, God, the Source, Mom / Dad God, or simply something greater than us. As we keep lightening our burdens, we begin to radiate the sweet sixteen or honeymoon glow.

Now, it is vital to distinguish between the two different kinds of feelings a person can experience. We've talked about the kind of feelings we experience when we "bite" into the poisoned apple and spin in doubt, which drains our life force. These feelings are created by an internal war. However, you can create a different experience simply by moving away from *The Wheel of Manufacturing Unhappiness*. Climb out of the ditch, accept where you find yourself, and hop on board *The Wheel of Manufacturing Happiness*.

Embrace the New Sensations

Another set of feelings may occur when you no longer "bite" into the doubt. These feelings/sensations are literally the old reactions and judgments unwinding. We welcome them because we know we are making space for unprecedented levels of happiness.

Yahoo! The old unsatisfying ways are leaving! Don't be disturbed or concerned with how long this clearing process takes. Keep feeding yourself with jolly thoughts, no matter how uncomfortable you may feel.

Let's consider another example. If you hear in your thoughts, "I am not beautiful," stop for a moment and listen to that doubt. Recognize that the doubt is there to remind you to love your essence. Accept how you are showing up. Begin to pump up all the "anchors" that make your heart feel extraordinarily happy, engaging your active faith by acting as if your dream is already a reality.

By riding *The Wheel of Manufacturing Happiness,* you begin to create something new, old programs begin to unwind, and the neural network in your brain is rewired. Think of it as reprogramming yourself. Remember that *The Wheel of Manufacturing Happiness* is spinning counter-clockwise, not in linear time. You are entering into the zone of limitless possibilities.

Think about how many times you have "bitten" into that same old hurtful pattern of not being perfect or not being worthy enough to be loved. For some of us, an entire lifetime of self-hatred, worry, and fear is all we have ever known. We may believe that we will never attain the beauty, success, intimate partnerships, or whatever our hearts are yearning for.

Let's consider the *Map of Choice* again. The feelings on *The Wheel of Manufacturing Unhappiness* and the feelings on *The Wheel of Manufacturing Happiness* are very different. The feelings on the left wheel are something that we are individually creating through our judgments and reactions. The feelings on the right side are simply unwinding the old feelings, clearing the slate, and opening you up to the new possibilities.

You may say, "Oh great. I've finally mustered up the strength to change, to become more joyous and happy in my life, and yet I feel like a train has run over me." Be patient as you release physical and emotional sensations. Remember, NO STORY.

One of our course participants did a "complete and delete" session, clearing a painful divorce which, although it happened many years ago, she was unknowingly still holding onto. She has wanted to get married again, but that difficult unresolved experience was keeping her from moving forward.

She went through a powerful "complete and delete" process and said that afterwards she felt the release of a lot of emotions. She even felt empty and vacant, realizing later that although this story was painful to hold onto, it somehow was filling a void.

As she was letting go, a sore throat came on. At first she felt frustrated. "Why don't I feel better from having cleared this huge file out?" Then she realized that repressed thoughts and feelings were coming out of her. She experienced a deep emotional release that she couldn't explain in words. She remembered not to engage or to try to figure out her release. She allowed the wave to move through her and afterwards felt a lightness; a burden had been lifted off of her.

As you let go of worn-out thoughts and patterns, be patient! Let's say you wake up in the morning, and your back is aching. You wonder what you did that caused the pain. What heavy thing did you lift? You wonder if you should call the chiropractor or the massage therapist. Before you do this, simply relax and repeat, "This is sensation. This is sensation." Say this over and over and over again as the old is "off-gassing" and leaving you for good.

The feelings are simply sensations. Calm down your thoughts, relax, breathe, and engage with the core of the sensation. You're looking to get beyond the label of pain.

A powerful "anchor" might help you through the sensation. Consider saying, "You are not real. You are not real." This helps to neutralize the fear and calm you down to allow the release to occur at a very rapid pace. In the movie, *A Beautiful Mind*, this fear clearing is vividly depicted.

"You Are Not Real" – John Nash Case Study

John Forbes Nash, Jr., after completing his PhD at Princeton at the early age of 20, went on to M.I.T. to teach mathematics for eight years. He dazzled the mathematical world, inventing the game of HEX, which was marketed by the Parker Brothers. Fortune Magazine singled him out in July 1958 as America's brilliant young star of the "New Mathematics."

Although everything seemed rosy for Nash, he developed a mental illness, later labeled as paranoid schizophrenia, where he would hear and see delusions, and was haunted by doubts and fears. He suffered for 25 years, often wandering through the halls of Princeton, seeing a child and man who apparently never existed. To him, these two people were real, until one day he realized that after many years of seeing the little girl, she had never grown. What a humbling realization for Nash. She was truly made up in his mind.

As he rehabilitated himself with the help and support of his loving wife, Alicia, he eventually returned to teaching at Princeton. While walking up the steps to his classroom, he saw again these two people who were to him as real as day. He said to them, "You are not real. You are not real. I'm not listening to you." Then he proceeded to walk to his classroom like a normal person ready to teach. He passed his test. He no longer believed these delusions were real. He pulled himself out of these delusions through his will and determination and went on to win the respected Nobel Peace Prize of Game Theory (the win-win business strategy).

From this example, we can see that if we believe in the doubts and take our thoughts and fears at face value, we are actually capable of making them real, whether imagined or not. We do not know what doubts were cycling through John Nash's head, but they certainly controlled him and changed his reality into a nightmare. John Nash's strength and passion for inventing new mathematical theories and his love of teaching gave him the strength to clear his demons.

Remember, doubts are our trainers. They surface not to haunt us, but rather to strengthen us, to help us get clear and to continue to hold to our dreams. We are NOT meant to get lost in the doubts. They are our friends!

The Surprising Balance: Your Doubt Level Equals Your Talent or Desire Level

What doubts are training you? Do you have your goals written down? Are you constantly acting as if your goals are actualized? Studies have proven that writing down your goals and dreams will improve your ability to manifest these desires by a staggering 85 percent. So write 'em down and watch 'em come around!

Here's a real-life example of a woman holding true to her dream of having an ecstatic birth. This example also shows us the power of transforming pain into sensation. You'll be amazed at the end result.

Ecstatic Birth – Corrine Bennis Case Study

Corrine Bennis and her husband were preparing to start a family, and as she learned about other women's painful, difficult births she felt there had to be another way to go. She made a choice to let go of fear and control and began tuning in to a wave inside of her body similar to the waves of the ocean. While birthing Jonah, her first son, in a redwood hot tub on her deck, she did not push at all, rather she kept surrendering. She said she felt like she was being carried and held. She turned the word "contraction" into "expansion." She felt like rippling kelp on the ocean floor, completely surrendering to the waves of sensation.

Although the birthing experience was very intense, she rode the waves and said she felt no pain. What was really amazing about Corrine's birth experience was that her son came out into the world still inside the sac. She never pushed him out; she allowed him out. Her water never even broke! She said the baby came out in an opalescent rainbow-colored sac in a very peaceful state. She remarked that by not allowing fear to come into the picture, natural endorphins kicked in, soothing the body, and anesthetizing the sensations.

As odd as it may seem, some women even have orgasms during the birthing process. They claim they're so relaxed, and they allow the waves of sensations to flow through them. They learn not to react in fear to the intensity of the sensations. For those interested, watch the documentary film <u>*Orgasmic Birth.*</u>

What an amazing example about transforming "pain" into an ecstatic experience. What are you ready to give birth to? Surrender to the sensations, keep the story at bay, and you'll move through resistance to new heights.

Let's review the two different kinds of feelings:

1. Feelings may arise when you "bite" into the poisoned apple of doubt and spin around the wheel. Around the wheel we go! Sometimes we can feel a "hang-over" and exhaustion from spinning in these judgments.

2. Feelings/sensations may arise when you are no longer feeding the same fear program. You are unwinding, "off-gassing" with "no story" and no need to figure anything out. Rather repeat, "This is sensation. This is sensation." Now is the time to strengthen your "anchor." You are indeed creating something new.

11 Fun Tips to Spice Up Your Love Life...

Here are some juicy ways to experience romantic renewal time during your busy life. These will deepen your relationship with your partner and create more pleasurable feelings in your heart and body, helping you to be *In Love Forever*. If you have children, have them visit a family member or a friend for the weekend (or visit a sleepaway camp during the summer) as you rekindle your love. We're sure you'll be happy to return the favor for your kid's friend's parents.

The main theme is "break from routine," renewing the love between you two. Even if you're working, create a fun nightly staycation or a mini-vacation. Discuss your dreams, interests, challenges, etc., and how you want the relationship to grow. The physical side will naturally blossom as you feel closer emotionally. Choose from the following delicious menu of tips:

1. Mysterious Lover

Plan a short getaway to a local hotel / resort for a night or two. Meet in the bar and act as if you've never met. Guys, ask her to take a stroll on the beach with you. Do your best to impress her with your romantic ways. Invite her back to your room as you gently slide your hand into hers. Expand your normal comfort zone as things get passionate. Maybe talk dirty or act out a fantasy. Allow your hearts to expand into more love as you pay keen attention to each other's nonverbal clues. "Oh... is that a knock on the door?" "Yes, it's a strawberries and cream dessert." Get messy! You've got maid service.

2. Take Your Time

When it comes to lovemaking, slow it way down, tiger. Create a playlist of love songs on your iPod or from YouTube or Spotify. Kiss, caress with your clothes on, massage slowly getting hot and heavy for at least 20–30 minutes like when you first met. When the fireworks eventually go off, they'll be more brilliant, and you'll both be smiling.

3. Top It Off with Chocolate Sauce

Cook a romantic dinner together in alluring lingerie. Have chocolate as the main course: macadamia crusted tilapia with white chocolate and coconut sauce or grilled steak with a red wine, dark chocolate sauce. Can't resist it? Go ahead and kiss passionately; remember, the kids aren't around. The sauce may end up on more than just food.

4. Play the Newlywed Game

Go to: NewlywedGameQuestions.com. The winner receives a relaxing, aromatic massage from your partner. No massage table? No worries. Place a few extra sheets that you don't mind getting oily on top of your bedding.

5. Reconnect with Your Closest Friends

Host a cocktail party or have just your most intimate friends over. Tell them how grateful you are for their friendship. Plan an outing together in the near future.

6. Kama Sutra – The Ancient Art of Love

Explore new ways to please each other and deepen your spiritual connection through lovemaking. Check out books and videos on this luscious, divine art.

7. Sext Him / Her

Send some juicy texts to make him / her feel special, such as:

"It's all about you tonight. May I take your order?"

"I'd love to rub warm maple syrup on your... I'll clean it up, of course. ;-)"

"Are you ready to feel safe and warm all night long?"

Many more sexting examples are awaiting you in Chapter 9.

8. Turn on Your PC

Squeeze and relax the PC (pubococcygeus) muscle slowly for 20–30 pulses. Start by doing this a few times a week and work up to doing it every day. You can be do this anywhere. Benefits include: more pleasurable, easier to experience and sustained orgasms for both men and women. For more information visit: wikihow.com/Do-Kegel-Exercises for her or wikihow.com/Do-PC-Muscle-Exercises for him.

9. Afternoon Delight

Come home for lunch and enjoy a quickie.

10. Make Her Think About You All Day

Leave a romantic note on the kitchen table or on the dashboard of her car, saying, "My love, I can't wait to look into your sensuous eyes. Be home at 6 p.m. Bubble bath, candles, and chilled champagne await you."

11. "Is It Okay?"

While lying in bed, ask your wife: "Would it be okay to kiss you?" She'll probably say yes. Then ask, "Is it okay if I kiss your neck?" She'll probably start to wonder why you are asking her these questions. Before every move you make, ask her permission. Wait for a "yes" before proceeding. Ask her: "Is it okay if I run my hands over your beautiful chest?" "Is it okay to kiss your nipples?" Then ask her, "May I softly touch her legs?" She'll start to get turned on more and more with every question, as you aim to please her. Hopefully, she'll try this out on you, too.

Creating this steamy (kid-free) time will assist you both in sustaining a juicy relationship (especially through the next few years, versus waiting until the kids fly the coop years down the road). Hmm, already excited about saving up for next year's sleepaway camp, are we?

Here's to being *In Love Forever.*

Call to Action

For the next two weeks, for at least 10 minutes a day, examine what feelings arise in your body and think back to the thought or judgment you "bit" into which created these feelings.

Please write out your observations in the space provided below and share them with your partner or trusted friend.

_____

_____

_____

_____

_____

Have you noticed when you don't pump up your dreams
that the doubts show up more frequently? Explain.

_____

_____

_____

_____

_____

What does "my body is neutral" mean?

_____

_____

_____

_____

_____

What thoughts will you pump in to transform yourself?

_____

_____

_____

_____

_____

CHAPTER SUMMARY POINTS

"The best love is the kind that awakens the soul; that makes us reach for more, that plants the fire in our hearts and brings peace to our minds. That's what I hope to give to you forever."

~ "Noah," *The Notebook*

- The body is neutral, a blank slate, waiting to be directed by your thoughts.

- Whatever you focus on, you create.

- When you "bite" into a doubt, you will feel "squirts" of feelings throughout the body.

- Your greatest gift to your child or spouse is your choice to be happy.

- A lighthearted approach deflates the power of fear.

- Use your imagination to create what you really desire.

- Let go of HOW your dreams are going to come true and focus on KNOWING they are on their way.

- Oftentimes, we are afraid to admit our fears, but by admitting them, they will usually go away.

- There is no room for hiding out in our separate lonely corners. Make sure each family member is clearing his or her space and pumping up happiness.

- All girls and women are beautiful princesses. Their genuine beauty is simply trying to bloom. All boys and men are grand princes.

- 11 Fun Tips To Spice Up Your Love Life...

- Watch the films *Lost Horizon* and *Phenomenon.*

- 90 day journey: Continue strengthening your relationship foundation from the first 60 days. By sharing your visions and dreams with complete support for each other, your needs and desires are being met. A deep love, joy, and pleasure to be your authentic self grows as your relationship soars to new heights. No more secrets.

Chapter 7

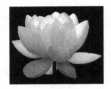

Secret 5 – Deleting Your Fears and Worries Forever

"You have a choice each
and every single day.
I choose to feel blessed.
I choose to feel grateful.
I choose to be excited.
I choose to be happy."

~ Amber Housley

Have you ever noticed when you are working on your computer after having downloaded many photos or music files that your computer begins to run very slowly? You may get frustrated and say, "What's going on here?" These files are dragging down the speed and efficiency of your computer and are taking up a lot of space and memory on your hard drive.

If, however, you choose to delete these files, or take them off your hard drive, your computer will start operating like new again. This process is very much akin to the "human computer," also known as your brain. Most of us have a few unhappy stories from our childhood, adolescence and even our adulthood, which continue to cycle in our thoughts and weigh us down. These unhappy stories become lodged in us as memories. As much as we try to forget these unpleasant moments, feelings of distress will continue to resurface until we have chosen to completely clear them out.

Most of us cannot even imagine living without pain, misery, insecurity, and sadness. We have become accustomed to a certain degree of misery, and, oddly enough, it can be frightfully exciting. Have you ever noticed that sometimes as you watch the news that you are pulled in by the unhappy dramas? Well, isn't it time to get excited about being outrageously happy instead?

Happiness Isn't Hard, It's Simply New

Have you ever considered the possibility of being genuinely happy all the time? Many people think such happiness is only possible in fairy tales, but The *Map of Choice* shows us that it is indeed possible to live in sublime lasting happiness, and it guides us with clues about how to move from unhappiness to happiness.

As we discussed earlier, there are two possible ways of approaching your journey in life: via *The Wheel of Manufacturing Unhappiness* or *The Wheel of Manufacturing Happiness*.

If you find yourself making judgments and simply reacting to situations around you, then you are spinning in *The Wheel of Manufacturing Unhappiness*. However, when you choose to stop reacting to circumstances and decide to utilize the "complete and delete" technique (shown in detail later in this chapter) to vanquish your unhappy stories, you will forever end the negative, haunting effect in your life. You are then ready to create your dreams while continuously living in a state of joy, love, and acceptance, spinning in *The Wheel of Manufacturing Happiness*.

While it's impossible to live in both wheels simultaneously, you can travel between these two wheels very quickly. If you find yourself in despair and making negative judgments, you can just as quickly change your route of travel by accepting where you find yourself. As rough as that decision might seem, if you put a different thought in your head, a positive thought of what you want, you'll realize that the doubt only existed to train you to think differently. Doubts, if reconsidered, remind you of the grand potential you hold within yourself.

We can't stress this point enough: Decode the doubt. The doubt you hear in your head will always be the antithesis of what it, your higher self, God truly wants for you. So get excited by turning the doubt into the positive (i.e. "You are not a good mother" becomes "You are a good mother"). Doubts show up to remind you to believe in your dreams, goals, desires, etc., and they will present the negative thought of what you desire to test your resolve in transforming your life. Why? To get your attention. It works, doesn't it? Then use the "Turn Your Doubts Inside Out" technique detailed in chapter three to quickly transform the feeling in your body. Something wonderful is about to happen by transforming the doubts. The doubts are truly championing you to achieve your highest potential by heckling you.

DOUBT scrambled is TO BUD!

If you've read this far, then you already believe that it's time to be done with some of those old worn-out patterns. By refusing to play the *blame game* and discontinuing your own *pity party*, you begin "**walking on sunshine.**" So ... what is <u>your</u> situation? What files are dragging you down? Perhaps your parents fought a lot when you were a child, you broke up with a past partner who had an affair, or you experienced a nasty divorce – and you felt scared, afraid, withdrawn, or angry. It's possible that you are still carrying the burden of these stories to this very day, despite the years which have passed. If you are, have you noticed that they are weighing you down emotionally, mentally, and physically?

Is this your family scenario? If so, did you ever consider that it was <u>your parent's choice to fight</u> and <u>your choice to react</u>? In this scenario, your parents allowed themselves to play out an addictive pattern of fighting and blaming. If they were to examine their thoughts before arguing amongst themselves, there was most likely a storm of doubts brewing inside each of them, maybe on many different levels, yet that storm was still there, contaminating the family environment with its sourness. As a child, these storms may have impacted you so completely that you never realized you could choose not to react in a fearful manner.

Take a look at your present or past relationships, and you may realize you are reenacting similar patterns that you watched your parents play out. The good news is that you can change these reactive patterns right now, so you'll never need to look back!

"Complete and delete" is a powerful technique to use when, and only when, you are ready to END any and all unhappy stories forever – no matter what your story, pattern, memory, or traumatic event may be. As you learn to end your painful patterns, you will show your children, if applicable, that they have a choice every moment as well. While change takes desire and great courage, you have to ask yourself, "What am I really losing by letting go of misery?"

"When you want something you've never had, you have to do something you've never done."

– Anonymous

Completing and Deleting Family Trauma – Cary's Case Study

Since I was very young, I witnessed my parents battling every day. Although they cared for each other, they lacked the tools to effectively communicate their feelings. It wasn't a pretty sight – screaming and yelling at each other, slamming doors, shaking the house.

I often would crouch in the corner on top of the landing of the second story staircase next to the only friend that seemed to understand my sensitive nature, our dog Beauty, a pitch-black German Shepherd. With sorrowful eyes, we would gaze at each other and turn down our ears as the battle wore on. My parents and three brothers never knew about this until I told them years later. I contemplated running away, yet I never did it. I guess I was too afraid. I carried this painful memory throughout childhood and into my adult life. I allowed this experience to affect my level of self-esteem and confidence.

As previously mentioned as an adult, in the effort to rid myself of this burdensome story, I sought out many different therapies. Some helped temporarily but none got to the root of my misery until I got sick and tired of myself and this gnawing memory. Even my wife, Wendy, was tired of hearing it. I remember Wendy saying that she couldn't believe that after 15 years of therapy and processing that this issue would still rear its head.

After going through the "complete and delete" process, I can sincerely say that this file of my unhappy childhood is closed and gone forever.

Soon after I did the "complete and delete" procedure I visited my parents at their house, and, as usual, they started to fight. I was in the kitchen when this incident was happening and when they finished heckling each other, my heart was open and I said, "What does everyone want for dinner?"

I was profoundly delighted and surprised to find myself not moved in the least by their arguing drama. In fact, I felt a feeling of unconditional love for them that I'd never felt before. I realize now that my parents acted as my trainers, and I had unknowingly hired them to "act out a role" and to push my buttons. By "completing and deleting," I realized that I am the only one who can either bring myself to or take myself out of happiness.

The pattern is truly gone and has never come back because it doesn't need to because I completed the test.

Completing and Deleting Lyme Disease – Fawne Frailey Case Study

For over three years, I had been in immense pain inside and out, bedridden, and on disability with Lyme disease. After many attempted remedies from Western to holistic medicine, I only made progress up to a certain point.

It was Wendy and Cary who so lovingly showed me that I had a choice – a choice to be healthy and happy! I was sick and tired of being sick and tired. From deep within myself, I chose to be done with my Lyme disease story! Truly done – not just small talk – but truly done. If and when fear arose about the disease returning, I welcomed it in as my dearest friend and reminded myself that I completed my Lyme disease story.

*Applying the principles of the In **Love Forever** system has transformed my intimate relationship with my partner as well. Thank you both from the bottom of my heart for your amazing work!"*

So the big awareness here is realizing we choose to react and make ourselves unhappy, and we set in motion a pattern which we often carry into our adult lives. In my case, when I was young and my parents were fighting, I didn't have the awareness or tools to keep me from being affected by their choices. I didn't know about the power of choice. But now, I realize that I have this incredible ability to clear my past and shift my reality quickly!

Let's unravel this situation and see how it plays out on the *Map of Choice*.

WHEEL OF MANUFACTURING UNHAPPINESS

Life Shows Up:

As a child, I witnessed my parents fighting practically every day.

Judgment / Good / Bad:

I judged the situation as bad.

Doubt:

"Why do my parents have to keep fighting? I feel very scared and unstable. What did I do to deserve this?"

"Bite" and Feelings Arise:

As I watch my parents fight, I feel scared, withdrawn, and angry. I feel very uncomfortable feelings in my body.

Stuck / Suicide / Substance Abuse:

Even at a young age, I may choose to end my life by committing suicide or may turn to drugs, alcohol, and/or food to numb the excruciating feelings.

Mask Over Feelings / Story in the Head:

I begin to dramatize this experience. I may carry this story throughout my day talking to friends about how screwed up my parents are. I swim in this uncomfortable story. How can I numb myself ? I need help!

Hope:

I visit my grandparents over the weekends, and my grandma feeds me comforting food, and I begin to feel relieved and better. Much later in life as I find these memories continuing to resurface, I go to therapy and pound pillows, getting out the suppressed feelings and talking out my past. I begin to feel better.

Joy and Trust:

Although the therapy stirs up feelings of my past, I am relieved to have someone I trust to talk to and this feels better, and I begin to trust the goodness of life again.

Trust Shatters / Feelings Resurface:

I speak with my wife about my relationship with my mom and express how I still feel so affected by my parents' fighting. I am mad that my past is <u>still</u> affecting me in the present. I begin to doubt the effectiveness of the therapy and therapist. My joy-filled life shatters and feelings resurface, and I feel confused and depressed. I have no answers as to where to turn as I have tried so many therapies already.

Now, let's imagine this situation from the other side of the wheel.

WHEEL OF MANUFACTURING HAPPINESS

Life Shows Up:

I witness my parents fighting.

Trust / No Story:

I may feel the old pull trying to get me to "bite" into their drama, yet I choose not to be affected by their fighting.

Complete and Delete / Feelings Unwind:

I do a "complete and delete" session witnessed by my wife. As I end this cycle in my life, my body feels an emotional and physical release, and my heart opens.

Pump in Your Dreams:

With every blink of the eye, I remember to pump in my "anchors" – happiness, sweetness, and the feeling of my dream already realized. Intimacy grows with my relationship with the Divine.

Enthusiasm / Inspiration / Creation:

Now I am in *the Wheel of Manufacturing Happiness*. I bring myself constantly to a state of enthusiasm and inspiration, which then leads to new creations that reflect this beautiful space.

As you can see from these two scenarios, these stories would still resurface no matter what kind of therapies I had gone through or how much journaling I had done. These painful memories would still show up out of the blue like sleeping demons until I cleared them out.

What is Your Situation?

Did you experience a traumatic event? For example, perhaps you didn't have a dad and lived with your stepbrothers, stepsisters, or a stepfather you didn't get along with. Maybe you weren't popular at school and were harassed or didn't get good grades. Have you been struggling most of your life with the way you look? Are you carrying an even more traumatic memory such as sexual abuse? Are you a war vet? With this technique, there is nothing too traumatic that you can't clear out expediently forever.

Can you see here that you have left your happiness to the whim of everything outside of you? It's time to start taking ownership of your life and your choices. It's time to think of yourself like a director on a movie set, directing many different teams – lighting, makeup, the set, the actors. It's up to you to get the situation and ambience just right for your film.

Similarly, it is up to you to direct your thoughts to where you want to go and to pump up your own happiness. If you don't "complete and delete" your self-defeating patterns, you will go through life in a constant state of healing. Healing never ends; it cycles forever like a never-ending onion peel. Like "Curly" from *The Three Stooges* says, you become a "victim of your circumstances, wawawa."

Cultural Pain – Case Study of Cary's Jewish Heritage

I come from a Jewish background. My paternal grandparents came to America in the early 1900s from Russia during a time called the pogroms where Jewish people were literally run out of their small villages.

Their story is much like "Fiddler on the Roof." I remember, as a kid, interviewing my grandparents in their apartment in Queens (New York) about their life in Russia. My grandfather's father was killed while being forced out of their village. My grandmother's father was also killed when my grandmother was still in the womb.

Every time I spoke to them about their past in Russia, they would only talk for a few minutes before they were overtaken by emotions and redirected the conversation.

Yes, their stories were traumatic and they never cleared them, so they lived their life haunted by their past.

Not only do individuals and families tend to hold onto painful memories but cultural groups do so as well. What I am about to say may be shocking to some, yet please try to understand that what I am expressing is coming from my own personal experience growing up in a Jewish community in New Jersey. This is by no means intended to insult anybody's beliefs. I have great care and compassion for the Jewish people and "the collective pain," and I want to see us happy.

My observation is that the Jewish people carry from their past the memory of being persecuted. One of the most important Jewish holidays is Passover, recounting the 400 years of slavery under Pharaoh's rule. In modern times, there was the Holocaust. Now let me be clear here, especially regarding the Holocaust, by all accounts, this was a horrendous experience. There is no denying this. Yet, we as a people, I believe, have yet to truly "complete and delete" these extremely challenging experiences and move forward.

Millions of dollars have been spent on building Holocaust museums around the world, symbols of the horror that occurred. By building such museums, we are keeping these stories and experiences alive in the collective cultural consciousness with the hope that nothing like this will ever happen again. But, unfortunately, genocide is still occurring to this very day around the world. So how can we move on from this place?

The first step is the realization that we are still carrying the burden of our painful past, "Oy vey." We may need to feel the hatred of those that have persecuted us, but we can free ourselves when we realize that these hateful people have been our greatest trainers. **Know that** no one and no thing has the ability to take you out of your own bubble of happiness. That choice belongs to you.

EVIL scrambled is LIVE!

Life is beckoning us to "clear" our past. It is relentlessly teaching us to wake up and create happiness. What's the harm in updating the Passover story, so we can learn from the experience and create a new, joyous chapter – truly celebrating and creating our "freedom" from the tyranny of our own thoughts?

What's so life-giving about holding onto these negative, fearful, disgusting stories? It's odd how humans almost enjoy talking about miserable horror stories. Remember, it's important to consider that we are passing our collective misery on to our children, with no change in sight. Isn't it time we clear this? It really isn't that hard.

Even in the darkest of times during the Holocaust, there were accounts of a small group who survived who said that just seeing the simple beauty of a sunset gave them hope for a brighter future. They chose in the bleakest of experiences to pick themselves up every day. They chose to live.

SCARED scrambled is SACRED!

Who is keeping our hearts beating? How many of us plug in our hearts every night as we sleep to make sure our heart charges up for the next day? In order to clear these painful stories, we must let go of our hatred for ourselves, our persecutors, and perhaps even the Creator or God. And although we may scream to the sky, "Where are you? Why have you forsaken me?" we must realize that God has never left us. We've simply chosen to feel alone, and we also have the choice to feel connected.

In many ways, the feelings we experience act as trainers. From the big picture perspective, humanity needs to experience life completely, including the mistreatment of others as well as ourselves. But we also must recognize that these experiences train us to feel connected to ourselves and our Source. The sensation of feeling alone reminds us that we have never been alone for one second.

Most of us have yet to realize that we can create genuine lasting happiness regardless of our circumstances. The realm of sublime happiness is awaiting all of us right now. If you simply desire it and take the actions to clear the way, you will enter your promised land in a blink of an eye. Like "Glinda" said to "Dorothy" in *The Wizard of Oz* as she was preparing to finally return home, clicking her ruby slippers, "You could have gone home any time." We can go home to our heart's desires any time as well.

The Influence of Unhappiness

Over the last couple of decades through popular psychology, we've opened up the closets of our individual and collective shame. However, because we haven't deleted these shameful and unhappy stories completely, their influence is still prevailing. Let's look at a few other public figures and their stories, which demonstrate how we hold on to our unhappy memories of the past.

Michael Jackson claimed that as a child his father physically and emotionally abused him, and he carried that hurt into his adulthood. Although millions of fans around the world loved him and his music, he was tormented by his past and his own self-hatred. Jackson most likely underwent therapy and sought out ways to deal with his torments, yet the point is that he never cleared these issues out completely.

Can you imagine the beautiful music and amazing dance routines Jackson could have shared if he had chosen to completely clear out his past and pump in constant happiness instead?

On the night of Michael Jackson's memorial, CNN's host, Larry King, was speaking to Anderson Cooper. He wondered how Michael Jackson's children would cope with the loss of their father. Both King and Cooper shared that they had lost their fathers when they were 9 and 10, respectively. King told his viewers that not a day went by without his feeling extraordinary pain and grief over losing his father. Think about what you may be unknowingly carrying.

I remember a colleague of ours asking her sister, a therapist, the following question, "How do your clients move forward and end the painful stories that they have so intimately revealed to you? When do they move forward? What's the timing?" Her sister had no clear, direct response other than saying that "healing takes time." But how much time does it take? How about saying to the loss or pain, "Whatever I experienced, I choose to completely clear out now. I accept the ongoing story of the circumstance playing out in my thoughts. You are not real. Thank you for training me to turn this emotional discomfort around by pumping in the thoughts of my dreams and creating happiness every second."

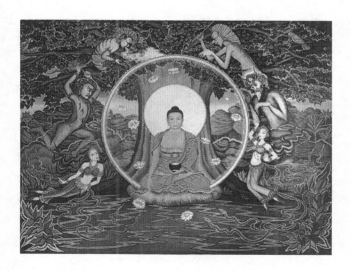

EARTH scrambled is HEART!

The intense pain and misery we each have felt is equal to the power, grandness, and effervescent happiness that is waiting for us. Inside each and every one of us is "hardware" capable of great love, similar to the capacity of love our Creator has for each of us. It has taken, for most of us, very traumatic events in order for us to experience rock bottom loneliness. We have yet to realize that these harsh experiences are here to open us up, so we can realize our true capacity to love ourselves and everyone else.

Each of us will get to the point where we will stop blaming circumstances and our persecutors for our pain and awaken to the realization that we needed these rough and tough moments to crack the shell allowing LOVE to pour out. With tears pouring out of our hearts, we will then go and thank our persecutors for training us to awaken to our love, for it was through their cruel actions that we learned to go through the full gamut of emotions from hate to love. These trainers reminded us to reconnect.

Ultimately, we have pointed the finger at our outside persecutors and blamed them for our pain; however, we haven't come to terms with our inside persecutors – those choices we made ourselves, self-loathing and unhappiness. We didn't realize that we hired these persecutors to get us to wake up and recognize the size of that miserable "bite" we took from the poisoned apple. How much fun are we having being miserable and choosing to feel we are alone?

We have a core human belief that we are alone, but it's not true. We are not alone and have never been alone, not for even one second. We are here to pump ourselves up every second of every day, to feel a juicy connection with our Source and everyone and everything around us.

Today is a new day. Now, you know you have a choice, and if you have children, you can help them realize that they have a choice as well. You can help them learn that they don't have to live one more second under the influence of unhappiness. If they ever hear a voice of doubt, remind them to reconnect to their heart and dreams. Help them understand that during adolescence, they don't have to feel alone, unattractive, or unworthy of happiness and love.

As parents learn to let go of their burdens and to communicate effectively, children will have role models who live and teach with sweetness rather than with blame and pain. We'll all be operating from *The Wheel of Manufacturing Happiness*, confident enough to explore and express our creativity with new inventions, new technologies, new music, new everything!

A new evolutionary moment is literally dawning, The Love Revolution – a new time upon this planet. And it's all so simple, so simple. It's simply a choice away.

Call to Action

"Complete and Delete" Session

Begin to explore an issue or experience that you want to "complete and delete." Journal if you wish, uncovering kernels of wisdom about the situation. Ask yourself truthfully: "Are there any more 'new' stones to turn over?" Do not rush this part. When you are ready to "once and for all" clear out this experience, it's normal, if you feel nervous about letting go of this "story." It's probably been with you a long time. The nerves are simply testing your resolve to "go for it" and transform your life forever.

When you are ready, arrange to have your partner, a close friend, or a neutral listener direct this session. Your partner/friend will ask you to reveal the issue / circumstance which you wish to be done with. For example, "I'm ready to complete my childhood trauma from living in a home where my parents were fighting every day." This is the time, the final hurrah, where you can bring up any last feelings about this incident. Take your time, breathe, and know that this is an important moment to honor the whole experience.

To Begin:

Your partner will ask, "Are you ready to complete this incident/pattern and never "bite" into this memory again?"

"Yes."

"Is there any more wisdom to be gained from this experience? Any more feelings to be felt?" (If the answer is yes to either of these questions, then make sure you clear out these feelings before moving forward, using the Turn Your Doubts Inside Out technique.)

"First, let me ask you an important question. If something different was to have happened, would it have? Simply put, did it happen?"

"Yes."

"Are you ready to move on and be complete?

"Yes."

"Are you ready to 'complete and delete' any association of pain with this experience?"

"Yes. I am complete."

That's it! The person completes the situation. It's important to note that very often, even as soon as the next day, you will be challenged with a memory of this trauma/pattern. Just say, "Hello friend. I have completed you. Remember? You can move on now." Be patient but persistent. Sometimes it takes a while to truly be ready to "complete and delete" your deepest and most challenging issues.

CHAPTER SUMMARY POINTS

"It is difficult for some people to accept that love is a choice. This seems to run counter to the generally accepted theory of romantic love which expounds that love is inborn & as such requires no more than to accept it."

~ *Leo F. Buscaglia*

- "Complete and Delete" is a powerful technique to use when, and only when, you are ready to END any and all unhappy stories, patterns, memories, or traumatic events.

- Doubts show up to remind you to believe in your dreams, goals, desires, etc., and they will present the negative thought of what you desire to test your resolve in transforming your life. Something wonderful is about to happen by transforming the doubts. The doubts are truly cheerleading you to achieve your highest potential by heckling you.

- With every blink of the eye, remember to pump in your "anchors" – happiness, sweetness, feelings of your dream already realized.

- With this technique, there is <u>nothing</u> too deep or traumatic that you can't clear expediently.

Life and the Divine within us are beckoning us to clear our past.

- We are now awakening to the realization that these horrendous experiences have always been our trainers, opening us up to realize our true capacity to love ourselves and those in our lives.

- Know that no one and no thing has the ability to take you out of your own bubble of happiness. That choice is yours.

- Watch the films *Life Is Beautiful, The Last Keepers, Faith Like Potatoes,* and *Brother Sun, Sister Moon.*

- 90 day journey: Any difficulties are handled immediately without a blowup or argument. A strong bond between you both creates honest, vulnerable, heart centered communications. Complete and delete any long term past issue(s).

Chapter 8

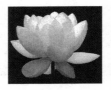

Secret 6 – The New Juicy You… How to Be Happy No Matter What

"Where there is love, there is life."

~ Mahatma Gandi

This is where the fun really kicks in, igniting the juiciness in yourself and in your relationship. As Michelangelo chipped away at his marble slab, grinding and caressing the marble, the brilliantly magnificent David emerged. What gorgeous essence is inside of you, waiting as you clear away the debris and judgments?

As you "complete and delete" the old stories and make choices that support your dreams, and support each other's, you're going to find, guaranteed, that you have more energy, more life force, more space to create the things that really move your heart. This is where it gets exciting, and it's worth all the hard work that you have done to get here.

Let go, dear friends, of any harshness. Let go of the old habits of needing to show up perfect. Allow yourself to be ecstatically happy, and then you will naturally feel juicy. Your "David" will appear.

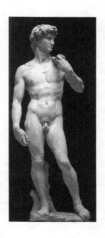

Honor yourselves for being brave enough to honestly answer the questions at the beginning of this journey and for the commitment to follow through. From your willingness to be more honest about such vulnerable issues, have you and your lover felt more sweet and juicy?

Perhaps you are single and want to get into a relationship, yet think since you have already been married twice that you do not have what it takes to have a successful relationship. Don't let the past hold you back. In those relationships, you didn't have a roadmap to guide you. With the *Map of Choice*, you now can have a successful relationship. You will learn to champion each other and to let go, step by step, of the harsh patterns. You'll learn how to genuinely love and care for each other.

The Courage to Be Honest

A woman in our coaching program said that she had a powerful crush on her yoga instructor. She called us on the telephone asking if we could help her get clear about how to handle the situation. At that point she felt excitement, shame, and confusion, all at the same time regarding her instructor. After all, she was already in an intimate partnership and was dearly committed to this person.

After coaching her about her situation, she gathered the strength to share this "crush" experience with her partner. Although her partner wasn't thrilled to hear about this crush, he was willing to go through his feelings and support her to get clear. She said that once she admitted the truth of the attraction she felt free. In the next yoga class, the attraction was no longer there.

Later, she realized that the yoga instructor emanated certain spiritual qualities that she was aching for her partner to also embody. Once she stopped trying to make her partner more spiritual and began to embody those qualities herself, her partner began to open up and deepen spiritually as well.

What Can Be Learned

We may find that when we are attracted to someone or something, we are really wanting to develop and express a part of ourselves more fully. We shouldn't be afraid of our crushes, but we shouldn't get lost in them or necessarily even act them out. By admitting our fantasies, frailties, fears, and jealousies, we become deeply open and honest. We free ourselves, then when we connect intimately with our partners, we are not just having sex, we are making love.

When a woman chooses to remember her sweetness and steps out of the judgmental shadows and fears of being imperfect, her heart ignites. Remember, gentlemen, your job is to make sure your woman's heart is turned on. Then, when you make love, her sweetness will help you turn your "hard-on" into a "heart-on." So, ladies, keep allowing the sweetness and happiness to blossom in your heart; it's like ambrosia for you and your lover. You will feel a reason to be alive that is so nourishing and, yes, sexy!

We all are natural lovers, and we already have the equipment and knowledge inside of us to be magnificent lovers. The difference is simply a matter of allowing your natural lover to emerge, playfully and joyously.

It's okay to "talk dirty" to each other; actually it's a necessary step toward a deeper heartfelt intimacy which allows your relationship to blossom, so don't be afraid of your primal self. You won't get lost here if you stay committed to the spirit of your relationship, so don't worry because you will eventually find a balance between your sweet and primal essences.

Enjoy the adventure together, you buckaroo. "Ride 'm, horsey."

The male/female bond is a yin-yang connection. The woman lifts her energy up, connecting in a deeply spiritual way. You might call this connection the Source, the Divine, the Earth, but no matter what you call it, when a woman makes this connection to her internal sweetness, she gifts her man with her heart while making love to him. He, in turn, adores her and the sweetness that she shares with him. And then, because his heart is so open, he gladly gives back to her and further opens her heart, igniting an even deeper passion. And so it goes ... the never-ending loop of divine juiciness.

When the man and woman are working efficiently together, there's a great sense of happiness and vibrancy in the airwaves. As a woman keeps herself clear of negative mental chatter, her heart keeps the man inspired, full of energy, and not bogged down by money and financial worries. Such a connected space is available to everyone, every moment of every day.

Wendy Reveals the Secret to Lasting Intimacy

So, here's the secret: When women open up on an intimate level from their hearts, their men feel their hearts open as well. The sweet woman's juiciness is the key to the man's connection to his heart.

In the past, I wasn't aware of how important it was for Cary to make love. I didn't put as much emphasis into our intimacy as he had and up to that moment had not realized how beautiful that connection really was for me as well.

At first, we were very attracted to one other, yet over time that juiciness began to dry up. I was self-absorbed about not looking attractive enough, gradually shutting down our intimate connection. Cary, in turn, was shut down by worrying about money and survival. We were fixer-uppers, to say the least!

After our journey through hell and back, we began to get juicy again. I'll never forget one night while making love, Cary vulnerably placed my hand on his penis and looked deeply into my eyes and said, "Wendy, the head of my penis is my heart." Then we looked at the head, and, funny enough, we noticed it was shaped like a heart! From some unknown place, tears streamed down both of our faces. While feeling the truth of the moment, we realized the powerful design of the penis and vagina connecting from the heart.

What I am talking about is not intellectual or something you can read in a book. This awareness came through us experientially. I also feel a profound connection to the Earth and her loveliness, something that we women can access and bring to the lovemaking experience.

Cary never seems to focus on the little things about my body that I have held as imperfect or unattractive. He sees and feels my feminine essence and encourages my beauty to flower. For a woman to receive such admiration and appreciation of her body from her man is truly a blessing.

Cary and I have shared this story with many couples and singles, and there is always a nodding in the crowd as people relate to our story, as well as a hush in the air surrounding the mysterious Divine Connection between men and women.

Many men agree that they feel a connection between their penis and their heart, and they often express that when their partners are not open to intimacy (saying they are too tired, not interested, etc.), they feel cut off.

Can you see why so many men end up divorcing their wives because of intimacy issues? They need to feel their hearts ignited through their women.

Do You Remember This Movie?

If you've ever seen the movie, *Cocoon,* you may remember the men jumping into the swimming pool and feeling rejuvenated and youthful because of the mysterious and magical out-of-this-world cocoon. They immediately wanted to make love with their women and took them out dancing. Think of your cocoons as thoughts, lifting you up, exalting you. Instead of drying up as we get older, we can become juicier. You have a choice to live in the eternal honeymoon glow. So, what are you waiting for? Let's go!

Make Yourself Irreplaceable

Here's a way to divorce-proof your marriage, particularly women. When you CHOOSE to be happy, feel juicy, and snuggle up to your man, you are making yourself irreplaceable, and your man will adore you for it. Remember that. And men, be the same way for your women as well. Know your value and be continually pleasing to the eyes and heart of your lover.

"The same way you got 'em
is the same way you keep 'em."

This enhanced level of juiciness in the relationship will open up new creative business ideas and hobbies for you. You will be inspired to discover refreshing ways to relate to your children, encouraging them to reach their greatest potential.

Note to Men

Can you imagine that just by having your lady behind you, encouraging your dreams, passions, and purpose, that money beyond your wildest imagination will come to support you and your family? Have you told your lady how much a rich, juicy life of lovemaking means to you? Have you noticed that when you stress out about money, or perhaps your ability to please your lady, that your sex drive wanes?

You are your lady's coach. Tune into her. Help her to stay connected to her heart. Help her free up the beauty and dynamic energy locked up inside of her. Compliment her. As you truly assist and encourage her to open up, you both will experience more juiciness, heightened levels of lovemaking, and financial opulence.

We all are born with the ability to be wonderful lovers. Wouldn't you agree that it is not about the positions? Although, it's fun to make love in fresh ways. Give yourself permission to allow your **inner natural lover** to come out, and you'll feel the ecstatic state of the "motion of the ocean" together.

> *"Behind every successful man is a great woman."*

Have you ever considered that the greatest ASSET you have is the woman in your life? She is because, as you assist her in assessing her sweetness, you will flourish in all areas as well. Your financial success and enjoyment of life blossoms from genuine lovemaking with your partner.

You need to help your woman become "great." **She needs your strength to help crack the shell surrounding and isolating her sweet heart.** She needs you to monitor her, making sure she is happy and feeling beautiful. You may not want to invest the time talking to her, rather you may just want to make love to her, but taking the time to work issues out and listening to her will be well worth it. We promise! You two will have earned each other's respect, and your dreams will flourish in this nurturing partnership.

Note to Women

When Wendy is not in a great space, it feels like I'm literally sailing against the current. Yet when she chooses to be in a great space, it feels like I'm gliding effortlessly. – Cary

Can you imagine what it would feel like to have a supportive man behind you, encouraging you in all of your heart's desires? Can you imagine the depth of love blossoming out of you because of his care and strength?

You are your lover's coach and manager as well. Are you tuned into what space he is in at any given moment? Do you know how important it is to be the wind under his wings and to support all of his dreams?

Have you thought about how important it is to your man to keep lovemaking alive? Can you imagine how beautiful you will feel by experiencing enhanced lovemaking?

Do you know you have the power to affect your family members? Ever hear the expression, "If Mama ain't happy, ain't nobody happy"? Do you realize that you set the tone for your home? Do you see how powerful your choices are?

Can you feel your essence, your beauty? Can you imagine combing your hair and discovering that it's silky, shiny, and lovely? Feel your beautiful feminine curves. Feel your lovely skin, your soft, smooth complexion. You are accessing your true beauty. Clothe yourself in the finest of fabrics that honor your loveliness. Resolve to NEVER EVER utter one more harsh word to yourself or another person again. You'll be forever a turn on.

Why not commit to managing your energy and wisely communicating without "biting" back? Why need to be right? Why not learn to deal with your feelings and live from a steady flow of love?

Sometimes There Is No Second Chance

We know of two couples who were in a fight, neither one willing to say "sorry," and in each case one of them died from a sudden heart-related incident. Don't wait to humble yourself and be wrong. You may not have a second chance.

On Jealousy

Part of awakening to being *In Love Forever* on a grand scale means coming to terms with jealousy, hatred and comparison, and all intensified states of fear. For so long, most of us, in this case women, have operated from an empty space, not connected to our Source, hating our bodies, and comparing ourselves to each other. We look for appreciation from external sources, are threatened by other women who may try to take our men away, and this kind of thinking drains our beauty. Remember what we said about a woman's power in the home? We have the ability to connect and fill ourselves with happiness, which nourishes our men and children as well. But we can also choose the opposite of this space – choosing to judge ourselves and to feel insecure and jealous of our men and other women at any moment.

Wendy's Struggle with Jealousy

In the past, I felt uncontrollable feelings of jealousy and suspicion towards Cary, especially when he was performing on stage. I noticed other women also felt very threatened and jealous of their musician partners in similar ways. I finally realized that I wasn't jealous of Cary. The jealousy I was feeling towards Cary and his gift for captivating audiences was representing the love I needed to give myself to allow my creative spirit to come out.

Once I realized this, POOF, the jealousy never came back. I finally passed the test. I needed to fill myself with the love and appreciation that I was seeking from the outside. It truly is a miracle. After struggling with jealousy towards Cary for so long, these feelings are gone. Completely gone! I can now whole-heartedly appreciate Cary and his amazing gifts on stage.

Here's a question you might want to ask yourself. Are you feeling jealous of other attractive women? Do you ever try to stamp out your partner's joy? Have you ever sent intense negative energy toward your partner because you are jealous of his talents? From your willingness to be honest, you can let go of these horrendous feelings. Again, what you are jealous of in another person is what your heart is aching to embody. Allow yourself to have it all!

As you become transparent with all these "behind the scenes" thoughts and unresolved issues, you will have exciting new conversations with your partner. You will want to please each other in refreshing ways. You might find that even after many years, you really don't know what turns each other on. It's never too late! Be open, like two little kids, about exploring new things. Have fun!

Learn to appreciate and adore your own and each other's bodies. Remember you look like YOU. You are a gorgeous human being. If you are not happy with the way you feel, change the way you think about yourself. As Leo Buscaglia said so well, "If you have big thighs, then marry a thigh lover!" Buscaglia would talk endearingly about his own body as being quite plump, saying, "I like my body. It's a neat body." Isn't it refreshing to witness such a level of sweet and endearing acceptance?

What's So Sexy About That?

To conclude this exciting chapter, here's a fun trick to try alone or with your partner. Try using the following phrase, "What's so sexy about that?" as a way to monitor what kind of choices you are making. For example, if you are choosing to work at a job just for the money, then your partner can ask you, "What's so sexy about that decision?" In other words, what is so life-giving about that thought or choice? If you are feeling fearful about anything – money, health, your children, your appearance – do you feel sexy? What happens to your sex drive? What's happens to your spark of life? Your brilliance?

Choose to Be *In Love Forever!*

Call to Action

Men: What are five things you can do to support your woman as she opens up and becomes happier and juicy?

1)_____

2)_____

3)_____

4)_____

5)_____

Women: What are five ways which you can be the wind under your man's wings and support all of his dreams?

1)_____

2)_____

3)_____

4)_____

5)_____

What are five creative things you can do together to enhance your juicy romantic connection?

1)_____

2)_____

3)_____

4)_____

5)_____

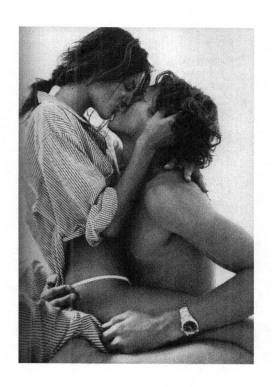

CHAPTER SUMMARY POINTS

*"The difference between an ordinary marriage and
an extraordinary marriage is in giving just a
little 'extra' every day, as often as possible, for
as long as we both shall live."*

~ Fawn Weaver

- Resolve to NEVER EVER utter one more harsh word to yourself or another person.

- "If you have big thighs, then marry a thigh lover!" – Leo Buscaglia

- Try using the following phrase, "What's so sexy about that?" as a way to monitor what kind of choices you are making.

- When a woman chooses to remember her sweetness and to resolve her tendency toward judgments, jealousies, and fears of looking or being imperfect, her heart ignites.

- Make yourself irreplaceable.

- Men, did you ever consider that your woman is your greatest ASSET because as you help her to open up and become juicy, you will flourish in all areas as well?

- Women, do you know how important it is to be the wind under your man's wings and to CARE and support all of his dreams?

- "If Mama ain't happy, ain't nobody happy."

- What you are jealous of in another person is what your heart is aching to embody. Allow all of your greatest heart's desires to be realized!

- Watch the films *Like Water For Chocolate*, *Cocoon*, and *Follow The Sun*.

- 90 day journey: Becoming better lovers than you both ever imagined. Make yourself irreplaceable.

Click the link below or go online to access more powerful tips on transforming jealousy at InLoveForeverBook.com.

Chapter 9

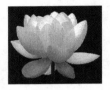

Secret 7 – The New Juicy, Vibrant Couple

*"Sometimes two people stay together
for the sake of the kids —
two kids who sat under a full moon
and pledged to be forever true."*

~ Robert Brault

Now we've come to the seventh secret – *Manufacturing Happiness* – the final step of this amazing, life-changing system. Hopefully, by now, you are beginning to feel the benefits of incorporating these secrets into your life, feeling more happiness, a juicier, intimate connection with your partner, birthing and inspiring new ideas, goals, and dreams. Have you grasped the life-transforming concept that you and only you can bring yourself to happiness?

This body of work was inspired by Rodgers and Hammerstein's *Cinderella*. This one-night-only, Broadway live TV performance, starring Julie Andrews as Cinderella in 1957 was viewed by more than 115 million people – one of the largest audiences in television history. A story of a girl who held to her dream of going to the ball, not only for herself but for all girls who dreamed. Despite many obstacles, she was unmoved, <u>choosing</u> to constantly live in a state of wonderment until she manifested her dream.

Are you holding true to your dreams and goals, no matter what may be in the way? Are you and your partner championing each other to realize your grandest dreams? In a sense, each one of us is a factory, and we all have the ability to <u>manufacture</u> happiness. Yet, in order to do so, we have to stop manufacturing unhappiness. When you begin to do this, you'll be accessing breakthrough power to create the things you really want.

Cheers to You

We congratulate you on becoming more transparent by incorporating this material in your life. Wouldn't you agree that it is a gift to reveal ourselves, especially to an intimate partner or friend/witness? At first, it may not be easy to be honest about expressing what you feel inside, but keep practicing and you both will feel tremendous benefits.

You will grow by leaps and bounds in an intimate partnership, especially with the *No Exit Agreement* in place. Being in an intimate partnership is tremendously rewarding, as it keeps you continually fired up about transforming yourself. Be it a child, spouse, parent, roommate, or co-worker, anyone can be a helpful trainer, encouraging you to open up to your fullest potential, so that you, in turn, can assist others in reaching theirs.

Doesn't it feel great to be shifting out of old patterns and keeping yourself pumped up with life affirming thoughts? Meeting challenges with a new refreshing attitude and transforming your old ways quickly? Are you feeling a constant appreciation for those around you and life itself? Keep practicing letting go of the clutch of fear. Consider connecting to something bigger than yourself, call it God, Mom / Dad God, a Higher Power, the Source, or Divine Mother. Whatever your beliefs, it does not matter. What matters is that you nourish your connection to the "bigger picture" with every blink of your eye. Have you been feeling a deepening connection in this area during the course of going through this book? The goal is to keep clearing and pumping in happiness, to be *In Love Forever*.

Let 'Er Rip!

You now have three highly effective communication tools – the *Sandbox Talk*, *Transcribing*, and the *Capsule* – to use particularly while you are clearing out the "muck and mire." Use the *Sandbox Talks* regularly to check in with one another on a day-to-day basis. *Transcribing* is extremely valuable in helping you sharpen up your listening skills. Keep the *Capsule* in your back pocket when and if your interactions get so hot that you need to let the steam out, all done in an appropriate manner.

In your communications, it's important to have a true desire to hear every word your partner utters, as well as to cultivate this attentive listening into all your other relationships, i.e. your children, business associates, and mother-in-law.

Every Interaction Is Precious

Stay present and desire to hear and feel the "heart of the matter" of what the other person is saying. If you don't understand, care enough to ask him or her to explain it again.

Always end your communication sessions with appreciation and respect. Let go of your grudges and the angry war. **Stop trying to be perfect.** Be willing to be the one who gives up the fight first. If the intensity becomes overwhelming, try using expressions such as,

"Hey, I'm sorry. Let's be friends again. Let's be lovers. Please excuse me for acting like a silly goose." You can even start whistling a happy tune like "Give A Little Whistle" sung by Jiminy Cricket.

You are learning to closely monitor each and every thought and to recognize when you might be tempted to "bite" into the poisoned apple of doubt and fear. Remember, the goal is to choose happiness, which will create a feeling of being in love. Constantly remember your "anchors."

You are living more and more in *The Wheel of Manufacturing Happiness,* where fear no longer exists, and you are living in a constant heartfelt state of enthusiasm, inspiration, and creativity. You are one of the first to machete your way to a world of happiness, making it easier for those who come after you. This action isn't based on anything external, nor based on a desire to have things go your way. It all stems from your choice to constantly pump yourself up with happiness.

"I live in the world of eternal joy and happiness, of absorbing interests. My body is the body electric, timeless and tireless, birthless and deathless."

– Florence Scovel Shinn

We know that the idea of everyone being happy may be a big stretch, but wouldn't it be amazing to have so many people walking happily, not because everything is going their way, just because they are choosing it? That is a wonderful vision, and it's up to us to create it! This is the end of the era of blame and victimhood and the beginning of a jubilant time on planet Earth.

"I think to myself, what a wonderful world."

– Louis Armstrong

Happiness Is Within Your Hands

Happiness, in fact, has always been in your own hands. What a new idea this is for most of us! It's exciting to know that the answers to our happiness lie within us. Happiness is an inside game. When we really think about it, we are our own best friends or worst enemies. It's always been up to us to change or hold on to crushing thoughts about ourselves, and these spill over onto our beloved partners and family.

Your life is changing as you are beginning to experience the effect of your own choice to be happy. Choose it every second of every day! Become a lover to yourself. Begin to fall in love with yourself and then with each other, living in a state of gratitude and grace. Step by step, you will become love and no longer demand love from your partner. All by choice.

As you feel lighter, both energetically and physically, you will have new refreshing experiences with yourself and your beloved partner and will live a more productive life. You will have more interest in yourself, your partner, and the world around you. And yes, you'll feel juicer inside and outside the bedroom. You will become a positive role model for others that are struggling to be free. You will take more and more risks to explore things that really make you happy.

Humanity as a whole is awakening to the realization that it is a choice to be down and out. No longer will it be sexy, or in style, to be unhappy and miserable. As humanity realizes that each of us has a choice to be happy, who knows what could happen. Maybe we'll still play and sing the blues, but we'll have more fun with the music and not be dragged down by it.

Maybe we will start writing new plays, movies, and books. Perhaps we'll create new inventions representing these new times. And maybe our songs will explore the unlimited possibilities of relationships that work, celebrating life and our Source. There is no ceiling here to limit what we can create and dream. This is an extremely exciting adventure!

Now humanity has a reason to change, realizing that there's a whole other world outside of the realm of misery, aggravation, and depression – a world of joy and unlimited happiness. Knowing there is the *Wheel of Manufacturing Happiness* gives us something in contrast to our present life, something wonderful that's possible. The *Map of Choice* beckons us to desire more for ourselves; it beckons us to remember that there is a spark, a lotus flower, born in each of us, just waiting to rise up to our grandeur.

THE WHEEL OF MANUFACTURING UNHAPPINESS EQUATES TO THE

D TRAIN *(4th Dimension)*

Doubt
Depression
Denial
Degradation
Decrepit
Disgusting
Decadence
Despair
Despicable
Dungeon
Death
Deadening
Dull
Disaster
Distrust

THE WHEEL OF MANUFACTURING HAPPINESS EQUATES TO THE

E TRAIN *(5th Dimension)*

Exhilarated
Effervescence
Excellence
Emanate
Exquisite
Elegant
Energetic
Easy
Everlasting
Enthusiastic
Euphoric
Exalted
Ecstatic
Extraordinary

As you walk down this road, you will feel and see changes in your life – real change, not just fantasy. Heaven on Earth and Ecstatic Joy have always been waiting for the time when humanity, individually and collectively, decides to say, "I'm tired of being miserable." Why hold on to misery, especially since you now know that there is another option?

The Power of Your Imagination - The Lavender Field

As Cary and I began to pull ourselves out of the cloud of misery, we started to have unusual experiences. In Idaho, we were the groundskeepers of an 80-acre wildlife refuge. During spring clean-up, we had the challenging task of pulling heavy water-laden kosher weeds (like huge tumbleweeds) out of the ponds in high winds and heat.

All of a sudden, we started to engage the imagination. One of us said, "Let's pretend we're harvesting a lavender field." We both got very happy, and the tough work became like play. We could practically smell the fragrance of the sweet lavender. Our friends even came outside to watch us and commented about how amazed they were to see us so energetic, despite being in whipping desert winds and dust. We were energized after many hours of hard work because of the power of our imagination!

Do you regularly engage your imagination? Have you noticed how you can quickly shift your space just by changing your thoughts? You can keep making this shift over and over again. As Tiger Woods has said, "Well. I did it before, so I can do it again." Happiness is waiting for you with every blink of the eye. Now that you know that, what are you going to choose? What changes do you need to make inside yourself to sustain such grandeur?

Options and the Fire of Desire

We used to think that humanity's only option was misery, but let's think about it with something more tangible. Let's say you need a car, so you go to a car dealership, and the only car you see is a used car for x amount of dollars. That's your only option, so you buy it. But if you had seen a gorgeous new car, too, for just a little more money, you would have probably bought that one instead. This is like our old model of humanity, spinning in the *Wheel of Manufacturing Unhappiness*. If you thought the used car was your only option, you probably wouldn't even ask if others were available.

But you know now that there are options, that another wheel exists, and it's accessible to everyone. The only thing you need is the **fire of desire** to change. And it's important to seize that desire today. While we may die 40 years from now, we could just as easily die tomorrow. But we don't just die, we will ourselves to death, and the same holds true about life. We will ourselves to live. Every moment that we live, life is slowly slipping away, but by embracing our happiness, we can stop worrying about death. We'll be too busy living!

Like Dustin Hoffman's character in *Mr. Magorium's Wonder Emporium* said, "I fell so completely in love with these shoes, I bought enough pairs to last my whole lifetime. This is my last pair." In the movie, Hoffman's character made a choice at some point that when his last pair of shoes wore out, it would be time to die. He admitted himself to the hospital, not because he was sickly, rather because he felt it was his time. He was happy, not sad.

You Can Have a Great Old Time Sexting!

Can you see the futility of being unhappy? In *The Wizard of Oz,* "Glinda" tells "Dorothy" that she could leave whenever she wanted. "You could have gone home anytime," said The Good Witch. So … what are you waiting for? Who is putting you in unhappy handcuffs?

What an experience we've endured. The wars on self and against others. All our atrocities have served us well by awakening us to this new dawn. Each of us is deciding when enough is enough. Phrases like "poor you, that's a shame, that's so sad" won't exist anymore. This is truly a new epic in the history of humanity. Let's celebrate! Let's literally and figuratively buy new clothes that best fit us now, that represent grandeur. It's time to come together in intimate ways with ourselves and with others.

And if someone still, after learning of this knowledge, starts playing out their old miserable "poor me, pity party" stories, their friends can remind them, "Come on, silly. Remember to choose happiness." You don't need to return to the painful stories in your mind ever again. You don't need to make yourself so small. Remember your heart and your dreams.

Do you see that as you hold your dreams and happy space that the doubts are no longer needed? The doubts only come up to remind us to shore ourselves up, training us to believe that our dreams are on their way. Do you need to constantly dig up a seed to know that it is growing? Trust in the power of your intentions; act as if they are already coming true. Let go of the nagging fear that your dreams are impossible. Live in the world of the imagination.

As your emotional intimacy deepens, the physical intimacy usually follows. Lovemaking will increase and improve, creating a growing feeling of orgasmic expression between you two. A sexy way to strengthen and maintain the juiciness in your relationship is by sexting (i.e. texting sexy messages) to each other during the day, especially leading up to a date night, the weekend, or a vacation.

To start off, you can send a text that peaks your partner's curiosity:

> *"Is it ok to tell you?"*
> *"Do you think you'd say yes…"*
> *"I've been dreaming about…"*

Once you start communicating back and forth, you can take the energy between you two to the next level by texting:

> *"I feel the best part of being with you is…"*

"When I get off work, I can't wait to see you, and..."

"All I can think of today is your..."

Once you have your partner's attention, he / she will probably ask, "So, what about my _____ are you thinking about today?"

Here, you can be cute or sexy by responding with:

"Your smell is an aphrodisiac to me." "The way you smile at me lights my fire." "How you look at me." "Your sexy body." "Your apple bottom." "Your firm butt." You can get even wilder if you want.

In this quick exchange, text flirting has begun. Have fun getting juicy with your partner. (For those dating, these same messages can assist in taking the connection to a deeper level.)

Now, let's jump into the deep end of the sexting pool.

1) Here's how to spice up an anniversary or notable occasion. Text your partner about a hot, past experience with him / her and describe how much fun you had and how turned on you were. This is a great tip for creating an endless supply of texting ideas. For example, "I was thinking this morning about the first skiing trip we took and how aroused we both were as soon as we entered the chalet. We made love in the living room. I still get excited remembering how sensually you took off our clothes."

2) Be more alluring, depending on how comfortable you are with talking dirty to each other. Feel free to let loose and use more steamy, racy, erotic language. We're positive you can do this. Here are some examples:

- "I love the feeling in my heart every time I come to your sweet embrace."

- "I'm freezing and need warming up badly. Let's go green and save on the heating bill tonight."

- "I'm getting wet just thinking of you inside of me…"

- "Hey love, I'm imagining running my slippery tongue all over your sensuous body right now."

- "Want to watch me please you?"

- "What's your fantasy? I'm your genie, ready to grant your wish."

- "Would you like to come to my special dance performance?"

- "Drop everything now, so I can show you how excited I am for you."

- "I got a new job today…surveying your sexy body, and every inch must be accounted for."

- "Sweet, pretty lady, you sure do turn me on. I'm coming home with your favorite take-out dinner. Dim the lights, okay?"

- "Dinner sounds fine, but I can't wait to taste you for dessert."

- "You're my dream girl. Come home soon. Flowers, chocolates, a steamy aromatic bath, and sweet dreams await you."

- "I want you to feel safe and warm … all night long."

- "Are you ready to take home entertainment to the next level?"

- "I can't wait to gaze into your soul when we make love."

- "Can you handle being teased until you beg me to ease your pain?"

- "How about a warm oil massage that will conclude with you smiling?"

- "I'm glistening, thinking about how I desire to please you tonight."

- "I'm thinking of you, and my love is growing."

- "I want to take you, my love … in deep."

- "I hear you're big and thick skinned…"

- "Come home and ring the doorbell. Don't be alarmed by who comes to meet you (just a warning), or are you shy?"

In summary, write your texts so that your partner is thinking of you in a positive manner from past experiences, or create make-believe situations which beckon your partner to write you back quickly because he / she desires to know more.

Talking about sexting raises another subject that is very important. Research as well as our own experiences in coaching many couples and singles has shown that many women experience temporary or long-term challenges with having an orgasm during lovemaking. The good news for most folks is that this difficulty can be transformed. As women, it's important for you to realize that for most of you there's nothing wrong with you or your partner.

Actually, the secret journey to more enjoyable, pleasurable lovemaking and orgasms is utilizing the following secrets, especially if you are having challenges: relax, communicate your desires and concerns with your partner, be totally present, and leave all worries aside. Explore new positions, stimulate and improve your emotional connection with your partner, keeping it fresh inside and outside the bedroom. Slow it down. Extend your foreplay. Break from routine, mix up how and where you touch.

Touch each other liberally from light (feathering) to strong, long strokes, and kiss (using your tongue) each other's body: shoulders, hands, fingers, arms, feet, hair, earlobes, inner thighs, buttocks, etc., Have long, wet kisses and look deeply in each other's eyes. Tease and massage each other's whole body before entering the erogenous zones. Both men and women report that taking more time has helped them feel warmed up, so incorporate cunnilingus and fellatio before your copulation begins, and you will experience deeper sensations and feel more love emanating from each other's hearts and experience yummier orgasms. Don't force it. Breathe, relax, allow, enjoy.

Foreplay is very sexy and juicy, and it creates arousal and anticipation in your partner. A Kinsey Institute study showed that 92.3% of women whose partners spent 21 minutes or longer on foreplay experienced orgasm. So for those that say it's stress from work, caring for the kids, or being tired that's causing the challenges with experiencing an orgasm, reflect on how much time you spend touching each other before making love. Let your partner know that his / her touch feels good by saying, "Oh baby, that feels so good," or by singing sensual moans of pleasure. Also, have the courage to tell and show your partner how you want to be touched. Foreplay has also been very helpful in reducing premature ejaculation.

An online article references McGill University in Canada and *The Journal of Sex Research*, and reports that the more foreplay you incorporate into your lovemaking, the more satisfying orgasms you will experience (Castillo 2014). Research in a study in the *British Medical Journal* based upon 918 men age 45–59 found that after a ten-year follow-up, men who had fewer orgasms were twice as likely to die of any cause as those having two or more orgasms a week (Smith 1997). A follow-up in 2001, which focused more specifically on cardiovascular health, found that having sex three or more times a week was associated with a 50% reduction in the risk of a heart attack or stroke.

In general, a lady's lovemaking engine can take up to four times longer than a man's to heat up and feel fully aroused. So, guys, take the foreplay idea to heart because once your partner's love oven is turned on and warmed up, she will be ready and desiring your sweet thang.

Due to the variety of comfort levels for couples in this area, we suggest you explore this exciting arena with your partner at a pace, intensity, and passion that makes you both feel comfortable. Here's a list of resources that can help you both greatly to deepen your lovemaking:

1) Kama Sutra and Tantra: These books, as well as many others, deal solely with enhanced lovemaking. Explore incorporating the spiritual side in the art of lovemaking.

2) Erosexotica.net – Tasteful, sensual videos showing how to create more pleasure for men and women. For a free preview of their videos, go to: erosexotica.net.

3) Sssh.com: A smart and sexy erotic destination for women by women utilizing videos, articles, and forums.

4) CherryTV.com: An excellent, insightful WebTV Show with regular women helping women become more confident, comfortable, and fulfilled in bed.

With Our Thanks

Thank you so much for learning these secrets and taking the actions in your life to make positive changes. We've seen extraordinary changes in our own lives and to see others taking advantage of this system and embarking on their own journeys is incredibly rewarding for us.

Our dream and desire is for you to be genuinely happy all the time. Our life is dedicated to fulfilling this dream. We ourselves have spent years building this Bridge of Happiness, sometimes flip-flopping back and forth from one wheel to the other as we were discovering the real meaning of doubt and strengthening our resolve to live in sublime happiness. The amazing breakthrough news is that not only is happiness possible, but you can look forward to a sustained level of happiness and purpose in your life with you and your partner, as well as with everyone in your life.

Please feel free to get in touch with us, as we'd love to hear your success stories at: WeCare@InLoveForever.com

As "Tevye," in *Fiddler on the Roof* sings so powerfully:

"To life! To life! Lechaim! / Lechaim, lechaim, to life!"

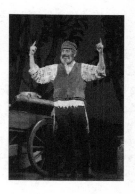

Call to Action

Art Activity

To sum up this system, this art activity will give you the chance to see and feel your choices at any moment. Once you finish this exercise, you may want to display your work to remind you of the power of your thoughts.

Gather a bunch of colorful crayons or paints and several sheets of white paper. Create a relaxed, distraction-free environment for yourself. Have fun with this activity. As much as you can, try not to think while doing this. Get out of the mind and into the body.

1) Imagine yourself in a judgmental or fearful place. How does such a fearful place feel in your body and look color-wise? Color or paint what you are feeling. What colors would be surrounding your energetic field? You may want to do several paintings/drawings. After completing this exercise, reflect on what

you painted. Can you see that your thoughts have color and an energetic effect on your body and that they also permeate your environment?

2) Now, come into a happy place. Color or paint what your happy energy looks and feels like. How would your energy look color-wise? After completing this activity, reflect on how your body feels when holding such thoughts and how this happy space around you feels as well.

Share your artwork with your partner.

Now is a good time to complete the relationship questionnaire again. When you are finished, compare it to your results from the beginning of the book. How much have you and your relationship transformed during the course of implementing these tools? On a scale of 1–10 (10 being the most), how much have you transformed? What is the biggest area of improvement? What area do you still feel needs attention?

Are you able now to catch yourselves when you're "off" and able to make the necessary adjustments, or do you feel you can benefit from having a relationship coach assist you in creating the quality relationship you are desiring?

Please turn to the last page of the book to
see if you qualify for a complimentary
Revitalize Your Love & Passion
Session offered by Cary Valentine and the
exceptional In Love Forever coaching staff.

CHAPTER SUMMARY POINTS

"Love doesn't just sit there, like a stone, it has to be made, like bread; remade all the time, made new."

~ Ursula K. Le Guin

- In a sense, each one of us is a factory, and we all have the ability to <u>manufacture</u> happiness.

- Maintain a constant appreciation for those around you and for life itself.

- Be willing to be the one who gives up the fight first.

- Step by step, you will <u>become love</u> and will no longer <u>demand love</u> from your partner. All by choice.

- It will no longer be sexy or in style to be unhappy and miserable.

- We will start writing new plays, movies, and books. We'll create new inventions representing these new times, and our songs will explore the unlimited possibilities, celebrating life and our Source.

- There is no ceiling to limit what we can create and dream.

- Explore sexting with each other regularly to keep your romance fresh.

- Foreplay is very sexy and juicy, creating aroused anticipation in your partner, and improves the ability to experience yummy orgasms for you both.

- Watch the films *How Stella Got Her Groove Back; P.S. I Love You; Shakespeare In Love;* and *Cinderella (1957)*.

- 90 day journey: Congratulations! You now have mastered this system, and you're on your way to constantly manufacturing a joyous, juicy relationship while deepening your divine connection.

Click the link below or go online to access
the Relationship Questionnaire at
InLoveForeverBook.com

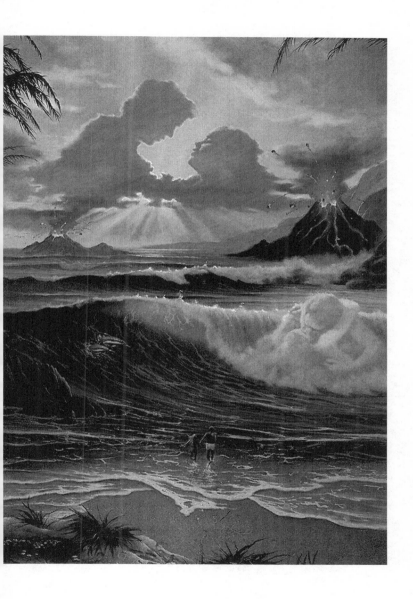

Epilogue

An elder comes to a child and asks him to explain what fear is. The child looks puzzled and stares blankly because he doesn't know what fear means. Then, suddenly, something comes to him.

Oh! I remember my grandparents telling me about a time when our ancestors used to live in fear constantly, which created disharmony in families and between countries. Unhappiness and war existed everywhere. Then our ancestors decided to stop fighting with themselves and each other and learned to choose happiness all the time. You see, sir, being happy is all I know how to be. It comes as natural to me as breathing. I've never known anything else.

Thanks to our ancestors long ago who began to change their ways and remembered:

Love is all there is.

In the future, as you transform yourself, your relationship, and your family, remember ... and choose to be happy, then we'll all be one step closer to this reality. Now, that's juicy!

Appendix A: Wheel of Manufacturing Unhappiness

This cycle shows how we travel in life when we bite into doubt & douse life.

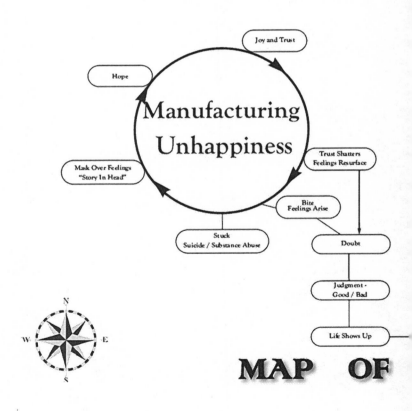

MAP OF

Appendix B: Wheel of Manufacturing Happiness

*This cycle shows how we travel in life
when we don't bite into doubt,
pump up our dreams & fire up life.*

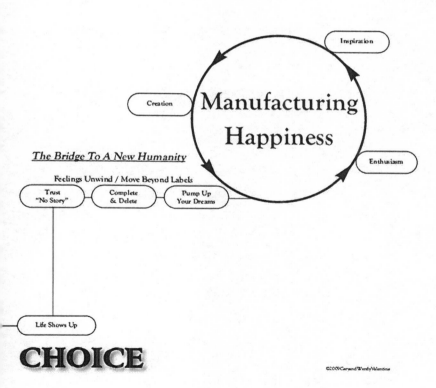

Appendix C: Map of Choice

*"Out of suffering have emerged
the strongest souls;
the most massive characters
are seared with scars."*

~Khalil Gibran

Imagine trying to drive from New York to Los Angeles in a car in the early 1900s. Could you imagine making this cross-country journey with no direct highway or clear road map? It would be practically impossible, and you would probably drive yourself in circles and bananas at the same time. Thankfully, as the years progressed, a highway would be completed which would make the journey quick and efficient. The road from NY to LA would not be built overnight. It would begin with one step followed by another, digging and digging, grading the road, until eventually resulting in a highway system which opened the world to commerce, tourism, and everyday convenience.

As in so many things we approach in life, we often find ourselves saying, "If only there was a map." Something to follow, which would guide our relationship and help us avoid pitfalls and problems. Until quite recently, such a direct route to sustained happiness was not available; we call it the *Map of Choice*.

After many years of hard work and commitment from our dear friends, Dan and Heather Jordan, this map was devised. Isaac Newton stated, "If I see so clearly, it is because I stand on the shoulders of giants who have come before me." We are so grateful for the tireless effort of the Jordans in bringing forth the foundation of this map. Subsequently, we spent years refining the map on our own and are making it available here for the first time ever.

We are very excited to introduce to you the vital foundational concepts underlying our entire 7 step system; these can be found on *The Map of Choice*. This map shows you the direction you have chosen in life at any given moment, based on how you react to situations. The map contains two different wheels or sides: The Left Wheel — Manufacturing Unhappiness, and The Right Wheel — Manufacturing Happiness. From first glance, we're sure you can instinctively select the wheel that represents the better choice, but it doesn't always go according to plan.

If we think about our actions in the simplest way, like when we <u>choose</u> to "bite" into any fear, doubt, insecurity, or worry which leads to unhappiness, we are spinning The Left Wheel (and Manufacturing Unhappiness). When we no longer <u>choose</u> to "bite" into those negative feelings, we are spinning The Right Wheel (and Manufacturing Happiness).

In our own personal experience, we spent a lot of time spinning in circles like a rat in a maze trying to find happiness to no avail. This *Map of Choice* was brought to us during a very difficult time when our life was falling apart, and when we were on the brink of divorce. Thankfully, after implementing the principles of this map, both of our lives dramatically changed forever. If you use these tools, your life will undoubtedly change for the better, too.

We will now demonstrate how all of us move in the map from one step to the other in the blink of an eye. Most of us do not even realize how quickly we react to life and constantly blame our outside world for our unhappy state of being. Since blaming is something we've done for so long, and often without realizing we're doing it, we forget that there is anything else to choose from.

Let's walk through the steps of choice with a real life example, while watching the results of the following reactions. At times, commentaries will be included in italics. Please refer to the map frequently, as it will help you understand the concepts as you progress through the entire system.

<u>Wheel of Manufacturing Unhappiness</u>

Life Shows Up:

I wake up with severe back pain.

"Life shows up" refers to anything or any interactions that may occur in our life which involve people, places, things, and often just ourselves.

Judgment – Good / Bad:

This pain feels very uncomfortable. I do not like these feelings. I judge and label this experience as bad.

We often instantly label thoughts and experiences as frustrating, sad, loving, hot or cold, loud or quiet, good or bad, or right or wrong. Whenever we label an experience, we are taking ourselves out of the moment and the experience.

Doubt:

I hear the following doubts inside my head: "This experience should <u>not</u> be happening! This is my unlucky day. Maybe my health is failing? It's probably going to get worse. How will I be able to do my physically demanding job and still support my family? I am already so worried about losing my job, and I don't even have insurance. All of our savings is going to drain away, and my wife is going to hate this and scream at me."

This is where the "blame or worry game" starts. If you believe what the doubt is saying is true, and "bite" into the poisoned apple of that particular fear, your life force will begin to drain away.

"Bite" / Feelings Arise:

I "bite" into the fear and believe that I have a serious problem with my back. <u>As soon as I mentally align with this fear, feelings arise.</u> I'm scared and must take an action to appease my fear.

Stuck / Suicide / Substance Abuse:

I have already spun around and around in this fear with my back for quite a while, and I no longer have any hope. In my despair and excruciating pain, I turn to drugs or alcohol or even decide to commit suicide.

Mask Over Feelings / "Story In Head":

I am now consumed in a story about my aching back. What could it be? Did I lift something too heavy? Maybe I have cancer. The pain is very scary and worrisome. Could I just be releasing emotions? I feel so confused. Help! I must get out of this pain. STORY, STORY, STORY…

Hope:

Phew! I found a great chiropractor that has helped a friend of mine with her back problems. I'm relieved and hopeful. I can handle this pain knowing that soon the doctor will alleviate and hopefully take it away. I'm calling right away to schedule an appointment.

Joy and Trust:

After a few sessions with this chiropractor, the back pain subsides quite a bit. My fear is gone. I feel a lot better and more joyful and really trust this chiropractor's services.

Trust Shatters / Feelings Resurface:

Oh no! After a number of weeks, the pain has come back. I'm angry, disillusioned, and even more fearful. Why didn't that chiropractor fix my back problem properly? Now what do I do? Blame... Blame... Blame in full force right now.

Now, let's use the same scenario and witness the effect related to a different choice.

Wheel of Manufacturing Happiness

Life Shows Up:

I wake up with the same intense back pain. I may not like the situation, yet I remember to breathe and not react.

Trust / "No Story":

I consciously choose not to engage my mind in a story such as trying to figure out why this situation is happening or seeking someone to blame for it. I trust that it happened simply because it happened. No need to figure out why. I choose to move beyond labeling the experience.

Feelings Unwind:

Instead of labeling this backache as "pain," I relax into the core of the sensations while repeating: *"This is sensation. This is sensation."* The repetition helps me to stay in the experience and allows my body to relax and release feelings. I remember to connect with my heart.

You are now creating a neutral space for the body to unwind emotionally and physically. Please take note: There's a tendency to wallow in the feelings at this stage and engage in a story. Constantly remember to guide your mind back to no story.

One little trick to break the tendency to wallow in a story is to "whistle a happy tune" or distract yourself with anything to break up the fearful thoughts. In this neutral space, take note of thoughts which rise to the surface. For example, underneath the backache could be long-held beliefs of not trusting that you are capable of manifesting all of your goals and dreams. Thoughts may arise such as, "It's impossible for me to be supported financially in my dreams. No one will be interested in my work."

As you let go of this story, you are literally rewiring your neural network, the brain's pathways that send messages throughout the whole body.

"Complete and Delete:"

My friend leads me through a "complete and delete" session, ending the pattern of not trusting in my abilities to bring in money from my creative endeavors.

This tool is used when you are ready to end a story forever that no longer serves you. The process is simple, akin to deleting old files that are bogging down your computer.

Pump Up Your Dreams:

After the powerful "complete and delete" session, I begin to consciously fill my body with expansive, blissful thoughts. I let my heart and imagination soar, acting as if all of my dreams are realized now. I feel electrified!

This is an exciting destination where you can begin to pump up your dreams and fire up your life force. Like filling up a bicycle tire with a hand pump, you keep intentionally creating a state of exaltation. If you stop pumping yourself up, your happiness will slowly leak away, pshhh. The concept of "pumping up" is vital to the 7 step system.

Enthusiasm, Inspiration, and Creation:

Through these steps you are building a bridge to a new humanity. This is the beginning of a new paradigm for humanity, living in a constant state of creative enthusiasm without fear.

Wow! Just look at the wisdom that can come from a simple backache! Isn't it amazing how you can have two entirely different experiences depending on your own reactions?

On the left side, there is only cycling and recycling in the same old pattern. On the right side, you are carving out a new path and a new you. In both scenarios you may experience feelings, yet on the right side you will experience the benefit of going through those feelings – more liveliness and joy!

Now, let's look at another powerful example of how the *Map of Choice* works. In this case, we will witness what happens when a woman judges how her body looks.

Wheel of Manufacturing Unhappiness

Life Shows Up:

I wake up and look in the mirror as I brush my teeth.

Judgment – Good / Bad:

I don't like anything about how I look. I think my hair is a mess, and I label myself fat and unattractive. I don't want my boyfriend to see me this way, so I quickly put on my clothes and go to the kitchen to brew some coffee.

Doubt:

Inside my head I'm thinking, "God must have made a mistake with my body."

"Bite" / Feelings Arise:

So many women look great. Why can't I look good? I hate myself. I'm ugly. I need to do something. As I make the coffee, I feel depressing, tormenting feelings throughout my body. I feel as if a sword is piercing my heart.

Stuck / Suicide / Substance Abuse:

I begin to pig out, quickly stuffing myself with donuts and cookies. I start to feel crazy and can't wait until my boyfriend leaves for work, so I can binge more. Food feels comforting and horrible at the same time. I hate myself. I feel like killing myself.

Mask Over Feelings / "Story in Head":

I've really got a problem, and it must stem from my parents' dysfunctional relationship. Both my parents drink and suppress their feelings. No one in the house communicates. I'm really pissed off at them for the way they have negatively affected my life. I've talked about this eating problem with my boyfriend, yet he doesn't know how to deal with this issue either.

Hope:

I remember hearing about the 12 Step Program, Overeaters Anonymous, from a colleague. She said the program really helped her to control her eating problems and underlying emotional issues. I think I'll go.

Joy and Trust:

I start going to the meetings, and they are helping me control my eating. I have a great sponsor who I talk to often, and she is helping me with a food plan and suggested that I work out my issues with a therapist. I feel a renewed sense of hope and joy about life.

Trust Shatters / Feelings Resurface:

Help! I'm out of control again with my eating. My faith in OA is shattered. The more I focus on the food plan, the more I seem to overeat. I went out and bought a carton of ice cream and several packages of cookies and ate everything in one sitting. I feel so fat that I make myself throw up to get rid of the extra calories from this binge. I even feel too embarrassed to see my therapist / coach. I look in the mirror and feel devastated because I look much worse than before OA. Now what?

This food issue has put a damper on the intimate connection I've had with my boyfriend. I don't feel sexy or attractive when I feel fat. I "bite" into the pattern of hating and judging my body over and over and over again until I decide I've had enough misery. I begin to direct my way to the right side of the map and learn a new way of trusting myself and appreciating my body.

Now, let's use the same scenario and witness the effect related to a different choice.

Wheel of Manufacturing Happiness

Life Shows Up:

I wake up and look in the mirror as I brush my teeth.

Trust / "No Story":

I notice my tousled hair and more rounded body. Initially I feel judgmental about the way I look, but then I take a moment and appreciate the beauty and brilliance of my body. I practice looking in my eyes and my essence without scrutinizing myself.

I still may not like what's showing up, but I take a moment to neutralize the feelings and focus on my heart and accept the parts that I do not like. I move from labeling to acceptance.

Choosing The Wheel of Manufacturing Happiness requires a desire, an "anchor," and a reason to change.

"Complete and Delete:"

I now recognize that the choice to be happy or unhappy is in my hands. I am ready to end this cycle of hating my body. I do a "complete and delete" session with my boyfriend, choosing to let go of my habit of judging my body. I commit to practicing unconditional love towards myself and to taking myself lightly. I practice, continually in my thoughts and energy, seeing myself as beautiful, rejuvenated, and youthful.

No matter what terrible actions you may have done in your life, or what harsh thoughts you may be carrying about yourself, choose to know that you are a gorgeous human being. Right here, right now. You may not look like a movie actress; you look like your beautiful self. Other people look like their beautiful selves. This idea of appreciating your own unique essence is well depicted in the movie, <u>Shrek</u>. When Princess Fiona finally dropped her human façade and became who she really was, an ogress, she and Shrek claimed their love for one another and married. Appreciate yourself for who you are and happiness will surely follow.

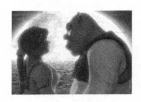

Feelings Unwind / Move Beyond Labels:

After the "complete and delete" session, waves of emotions, memories, and physical sensations arise. I remember that I chose "No Story" to calm myself down, and I begin repeating the phrases: "This is sensation. This is sensation," and it allows me to release my negative thoughts. Although it may not feel like it at the time, these uncomfortable feelings are a gift, as the old harsh behaviors are leaving.

226

At times I feel tempted to look in the mirror from a scrutinizing place, yet I remember to turn the doubt inside out and feel my beauty. I use my "anchor" to strengthen my resolve to end this pattern. If this subject comes up again, I say, "Thank you. I've already completed you."

Pump Up Your Dreams:

I feel freed up and more and more energized as inspiring ideas flow through me. I am now actually manufacturing happiness bricks instead of manufacturing unhappiness bricks and can start focusing on things that make my heart merry.

Most of us have become addicted to the left side of this map and unknowingly have cycled continuously around the wheel feeling depleted, depressed, lonely, and passionless. This cycling will lead us nowhere new. Let's learn a new way to play the game of life by slamming on our brakes and refusing to "bite" into the same "poisoned apple." Each time we refuse the temptation, our purpose and reason to live becomes mightier.

Oftentimes, in order to make change, you may need what we call an "anchor" – a reason or something that's bigger than yourself. Be it your children, your main relationship, or a dream. Or maybe it is pain that's motivating you. Whatever your reason to change is, may this *Map of Choice* be a guiding force on your journey.

The map is something to come back to time and time again, guiding you as situations show up. Keep reviewing your life and examining how your choices play out on the map until you have memorized all the destination stops and are living your life entirely from the right side of the map. Each time you make a choice to shift out of fear, you are taking the next step in building a bridge to a new humanity. Have fun examining your choices and allow this map to become a great friend.

At first, you may feel pressured to understand these concepts, but you don't need to hurry. It certainly took us a long time to realize the steps on this map. Give yourself the permission and freedom to allow the wisdom to unfold naturally. It may not all make sense initially, but it will over time. And if you keep coming back to these ideas (of being responsible for creating your own happiness or unhappiness), then as you read the material, you will begin putting yourself and your experiences on the map. Then the map will have value for you.

Did You Notice …

Please note that on the left wheel of the map, the arrows are moving in a <u>clockwise</u> motion, signifying that you are moving in linear time, creating the same old misery. On the right wheel, the arrows are moving <u>counterclockwise,</u> signifying that you are moving out of time, creating something entirely new.

Call to Action

Map out your reactions using the concepts from the Wheel of Manufacturing Unhappiness by answering the question associated with each heading below, then write out your new perspective using the concepts from the Wheel of Manufacturing Happiness. By completing this exercise, you will ground the critically important idea of choice in every second of your life.

Wheel of Manufacturing Unhappiness

Life Shows Up: (How is life showing up?)

_____

_____

_____

_____

Judgment – Good / Bad: (How are you judging this situation?)

_____

_____

_____

_____

Doubt: (Do you feel this situation should not be happening?)

_____

_____

_____

_____

"Bite" / Feelings Arise: (What happens when you "bite" into the fear?)

_____

_____

_____

_____

Stuck / Suicide / Substance Abuse: (Are you turning to alcohol, sex, or drugs to mask over the feelings? Have you considered suicide?)

_____

_____

_____

_____

Mask Over Feelings / "Story in Head": (What story is going through your head?)

_____

_____

_____

_____

Hope: (Have you found a hopeful solution to your problem?)

_____
_____
_____
_____

Joy and Trust: (Has this solution created trust and joy in your life?)

_____
_____
_____
_____

Trust Shatters / Feelings Resurface: (Have the feelings returned?)

_____
_____
_____
_____

<u>Wheel Of Manufacturing Happiness</u>

Life Shows Up: (How is life showing up?)

_____

_____

_____

_____

Trust / "No Story": (Are you remembering to put in an "anchor" and not to engage in a story?)

_____

_____

_____

_____

"Complete and Delete:" (Have you gone through a "complete and delete" session regarding this issue?)

_____

_____

_____

_____

Feelings Unwind: (Are you remembering to repeat, "This is sensation" to yourself?)

_____

_____

_____

_____

Pump Up Your Dreams: (What dreams are you pumping up?)

_____

_____

_____

_____

Enthusiasm, Inspiration, Creation: (What new ideas are being conceived?)

_____

_____

_____

_____

CHAPTER SUMMARY POINTS

"We love because it's the only true adventure."

~Nikki Giovanni

- You have a choice, every second, to be happy or unhappy.

- Break the habit of negative thinking and reacting.

- Stop the loop of drama and negative thinking. Opt for "No Story."

- Constantly pump yourself up with exalting thoughts and powerful visions, creating a new you, a new relationship, and a new humanity.

- Allow the old thoughts and patterns to unwind by saying, "This is sensation," or "feelings are my friends."

- Change the way you label experiences from, "I'm in pain," to "I'm feeling a lot of sensation." Relax, allow the feelings to release, and allow your heart to open.

- Cultivate an "anchor," a mantra, or a strong enough reason to transform yourself.

- Do a "complete and delete" session when you are ready to end a story that no longer serves you – forever.

- Use the *Map of Choice* as your foundation, and come back to it time and time again. It will help you remember not to judge and to constantly pump up your dreams.

- Watch the films *The Legend of Bagger Vance* and *Field of Dreams*.

Appendix D: Movie Recommendations

Inspirational

American President
Apollo 13
Beautiful Dreamers
Brother Sun, Sister Moon
Can't Take It With You
Cinderella (Julie Andrews - PBS, 1957)
Coach Carter
Cocoon
Dances with Wolves
Defending Your Life
Endurance (PBS)
Faith Like Potatoes
Fern Gully

Field of Dreams
Fire Proof
It's a Beautiful Life
Jesus of Nazareth
Little Buddha
Lord of the Rings
Love Is All You Need
Lost Horizon
Mama Mia!
Mary Poppins
Miracle on 34th Street
Mr. Magorium's Wonder Emporium
October Sky
Orgasmic Birth (Documentary)
Pollyanna
P.S. I Love You
Renaissance Man
Rocky
The Father Damien Story
The Man Who Planted Trees
Titanic

<u>Stepping Out of Doubt and Fear</u>

Arthur
Aladdin
Beautiful Mind
Children of a Lesser God
Condition Black
Dead Poets Society
Defending Your Life
Follow the Sun
Harvey
It's a Wonderful Life
Jerry Maguire
Karate Kid
Lean On Me
Les Misérables (1998)
Like Water for Chocolate
Little Mermaid
Man On Wire
Meet the Fockers
Mississippi Masala
Monsters, Inc.
Mr. Smith Goes to Washington
Saving Mr. Banks
Scrooge (Albert Finney)
Shakespeare In Love
Shrek
Snow White
Stand and Deliver
The American President

The Bodyguard
The Incredibles
The Last Keepers
The Legend of Bagger Vance
The Matrix
Touching the Void
When a Man Loves a Woman
Wizard of Oz

Appendix E: Love Songs

This is a sampling of love songs from different eras. What's your wedding or love song? Surprise your partner and play it on special occasions.

A Thousand Years – Christina Perri
All I Want For Christmas Is You – Mariah Carey
At Last – Eva Cassidy
Biggest Part of Me – Ambrosia
Can't Help Falling In Love – Elvis Presley
Cheek to Cheek – Fred Astaire
Endless Love – Lionel Richie & Diana Ross
Everything – Michael Bublé
For Once in My Life – Frank Sinatra
From This Moment On – Shania Twain
Have You Ever Really Loved a Woman – Bryan Adams
I Believe In You and Me – Whitney Houston

Islands in the Stream – Bee Gees
L.O.V.E. – Nat King Cole
La Vie En Rose – Edith Piaf
La Voce del Silenzio – Andrea Bocelli
Lady in Red – Chris de Burgh
Marry Me – Train
Marry You – Bruno Mars
My Heart Will Go On – Celine Dion
Never Gonna Be Alone – Nickelback
Something – Beatles
Stand By Me – Ben E. King
The First Time Ever I Saw Your Face – Jeffrey Gaines
Un Amor – Gypsy Kings
Unchained Melody – The Righteous Brothers
You and Me – Lifehouse
You Are the Sunshine of My Life – Stevie Wonder

Appendix F: *New York Times* Article – Is Marriage Good for Your Health?

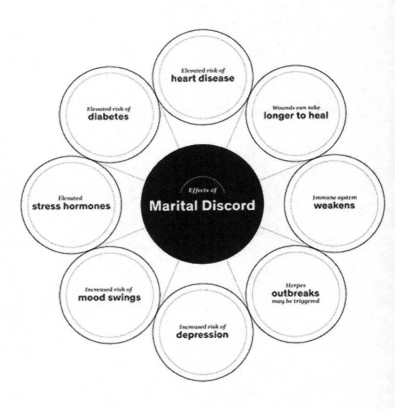

April 14, 2010

𝕺𝖍𝖊 𝕹𝖊𝖜 𝖄𝖔𝖗𝖐 𝕿𝖎𝖒𝖊𝖘

Is Marriage Good for Your Health?

By TARA PARKER-POPE

In 1858, a British epidemiologist named William Farr set out to study what he called the "conjugal condition" of the people of France. He divided the adult population into three distinct categories: the "married," consisting of husbands and wives; the "celibate," defined as the bachelors and spinsters who had never married; and finally the "widowed," those who had experienced the death of a spouse. Using birth, death and marriage records, Farr analyzed the relative mortality rates of the three groups at various ages. The work, a groundbreaking study that helped establish the field of medical statistics, showed that the unmarried died from disease "in undue proportion" to their married counterparts. And the widowed, Farr found, fared worst of all.

Farr's was among the first scholarly works to suggest that there is a health advantage to marriage and to identify marital loss as a significant risk factor for poor health. Married people, the data seemed to show, lived longer, healthier lives. "Marriage is a healthy estate," Farr concluded. "The single individual is more likely to be wrecked on his voyage than the lives joined together in matrimony."

While Farr's own study is no longer relevant to the social realities of today's world — his three categories exclude couples living together, gay couples and the divorced, for instance — his overarching finding about the health benefits of marriage seems to have stood the test of time. Critics, of course, have rightly cautioned about the risk of conflating correlation with causation. (Better health among the married sometimes simply reflects the fact that healthy people are more likely to get married in the first place.) But in the 150 years since Farr's work, scientists have continued to document the "marriage advantage": the fact that married people, on average, appear to be healthier and live longer than unmarried people.

Contemporary studies, for instance, have shown that married people are less likely to get pneumonia, have surgery, develop cancer or have heart attacks. A group of Swedish researchers has found that being married or cohabiting at midlife is associated with a lower risk for dementia. A study of two dozen causes of death in the Netherlands found that in virtually every category, ranging from violent deaths like homicide and car accidents to certain forms of cancer, the unmarried were at far higher risk than the married. For many years, studies like these have influenced both politics and policy, fueling national marriage-promotion efforts, like the Healthy Marriage Initiative of the U.S. Department of Health and Human Services. From 2006 to 2010, the program received

$150 million annually to spend on projects like "divorce reduction" efforts and often cited the health benefits of marrying and staying married.

But while it's clear that marriage is profoundly connected to health and well-being, new research is increasingly presenting a more nuanced view of the so-called marriage advantage. Several new studies, for instance, show that the marriage advantage doesn't extend to those in troubled relationships, which can leave a person far less healthy than if he or she had never married at all. One recent study suggests that a stressful marriage can be as bad for the heart as a regular smoking habit. And despite years of research suggesting that single people have poorer health than those who marry, a major study released last year concluded that single people who have never married have better health than those who married and then divorced.

All of which suggests that while Farr's exploration into the conjugal condition pointed us in the right direction, it exaggerated the importance of the institution of marriage and underestimated the quality and character of the marriage itself. The mere fact of being married, it seems, isn't enough to protect your health. Even the Healthy Marriage Initiative makes the distinction between "healthy" and "unhealthy" relationships when discussing the benefits of marriage. "When we divide good marriages from bad ones," says the marriage historian Stephanie Coontz, who is also the director of research and public education for the Council on Contemporary

Families, "we learn that it is the relationship, not the institution, that is key."

Some of today's most interesting research on the relationship between marriage and health is being led by a pair of researchers at Ohio State University College of Medicine. The duo, Ronald Glaser and Jan Kiecolt-Glaser, are also, fittingly, married to each other.

Glaser and Kiecolt-Glaser's scholarly collaboration has its roots in a chance encounter during a faculty picnic in October 1978 on the Ohio State campus. Glaser, who is a viral immunologist, spotted an attractive woman standing with members of the psychiatry faculty. Although their eyes met only briefly, he caught a glimpse of her name tag. Intrigued, he tried to track her down, calling the psychiatry department chairman to ask if he knew a petite blonde on staff with a name like "Pam Kiscoli." The department chairman figured out that Glaser was talking about a new assistant professor named Jan Kiecolt. Glaser and Kiecolt eventually met for lunch at the university's hospital cafeteria. They married a year later, in January 1980.

The coupling resulted in more than romance. The two scientists were fascinated by each other's work, which they often discussed over meals or while jogging together. Glaser suggested that they collaborate professionally, but finding common ground was a challenge: he studied virology and immunology; she was a clinical psychologist who focused on assertiveness and other behavior. In the early 1980s, however, Kiecolt-Glaser came across a book on the emerging field of psychoneuroimmunology, which concerns the interplay between behavior, the immune and endocrine systems and the brain and nervous system. The couple were intrigued by a science that lay at the intersection of their disciplines. Today, the two disagree on exactly how their professional collaboration began. "He says I started it," Kiecolt-Glaser told me. "But I say he started it."

In their first research collaboration, they sought to measure the effect of psychological stress on the immune system. Although earlier studies had established that trauma and other major stress — like the death of a loved one or prolonged sleep deprivation — weakened the immune system, the Glasers wanted to know if lesser forms of stress, like those associated with the workplace or graduate school, had a similar effect.

The Glasers, who worked at Ohio's State's medical school, had ready access to an ample supply of stressed-out students, and so they decided to study the toll exacted by school pressure. They took blood samples from a set of students early in the semester and then did so again in the middle of final exams. The Glasers discovered that the stress of examination time seemed to cause a significant weakening of the students' immune response: by examination time, the medical students showed a significant drop in so-called natural killer cells, a type of white blood cell that battles viruses and helps prevent cancer.

For their second collaboration, the Glasers turned their attention to domestic strife. They wondered about the role that relationships play in health and about the effects of marital stress, which, like school pressure, can be a source of nontraumatic but chronic strain. In what was to be the first of their many studies on marriage and health, the Glasers recruited 76 women, half of whom were married; the other half were separated or had divorced. The Glasers wanted to identify which married women were in troubled relationships as well as which of the women who were separated or divorced from their husbands were emotionally struggling the most. They did this by using marital-quality scales, types of questionnaires that ask couples to indicate agreement or disagreement with statements like "If I had to do it over again, I would marry the same person" or "We often do things together." Next, using blood tests, the Glasers measured the women's immune-system responses, tracking their levels of antibody production and other indicators of immunity strength. The results showed that the women in unhappy relationships and the women who remained emotionally hung up on their ex-husbands had decidedly weaker immune responses than the women who were in happier relationships (or were happily out of them).

Though pleased with this study, the Glasers knew that they had succeeded in taking the measure of marital happiness and health only at a single moment. The couple were also curious to study the effect of marital stress as it unfolded in real time. What happens to the body minute by minute, hour by hour, when couples engage in hostile marital disputes? To find this out, they recruited a study group of 90 seemingly happy newlywed couples. Each couple was hooked up to tubes so that blood samples could be drawn from the pair at regular intervals, and the husband and wife were seated face to face. Obscured by a curtain, the researchers watched the couples on video monitors; nurses took the blood samples. The participants, as they had been prompted to do, discussed their most volatile topics of marital conflict, like housework, sex or interference from a mother-in-law. "You wouldn't think in a study situation that they would tear into each other," Glaser, who is now the director of the Institute for Behavioral Medicine Research, told me. "But they get into it." As expected, the couples who exhibited the most negative and hostile behavior during the conflict discussion showed the largest declines in immune-system function during the 24-hour study period.

These data strongly suggested that marital stress could affect the body in striking ways, but the Glaser team had yet to prove that marital conflict had any truly meaningful or lasting effect on health. Kiecolt-Glaser had an idea for another study that would meet this higher standard. She had read about a strange tool used by her dermatology colleagues: a small plastic suction device designed to leave eight tiny blisters on the arm and allow monitoring of the immune-system response at the wound sites. Kiecolt-Glaser's proposal was to use this blistering device to measure how quickly or slowly physical wounds healed among married couples who had undergone different levels of marital stress.

The experiment had two phases. Each married couple, after their forearms were subjected to the blistering procedure, were asked to talk together for a half-hour: on one occasion they discussed topics chosen to elicit the couples' supportive behaviors; on another day, after undergoing the blistering procedures again, they discussed topics selected to evoke conflict and tension and tried to resolve them. Before subjecting others to the blistering regimen, each of the Glasers had the device secured to his or her respective forearm to have his or her skin blistered. The sensation is comparable to "someone gently pinching your arm," Kiecolt-Glaser told me. Nonetheless, the Glasers knew it would be a tough sell to convince others couples to undergo the blistering procedure as well as two weeks of subsequent monitoring of the wounds as they healed. A study grant allowed them to offer $2,000 in total compensation to any couple willing to take part in the experiment. They managed to recruit 42 married couples for the study.

The results were remarkable. After the blistering sessions in which couples argued, their wounds took, on average, a full day longer to heal than after the sessions in which the couples discussed something pleasant. Among couples who exhibited especially high levels of hostility while bickering, the wounds took a full two days longer to heal than those of couples who had showed less animosity while fighting.

Published in 2005 in The Archives of General Psychiatry, the Glasers' findings help explain epidemiological data showing that couples in troubled marriages appear to be more susceptible to illness than happier couples. The results may also have practical relevance for surgical patients, for instance, waiting for incisions to heal. But most important, the study offered compelling evidence that a hostile fight with your husband or wife isn't just bad for your relationship. It can have a profound toll on your body.

Kiecolt-Glaser told me that the overall health lesson to take away from the new wave of marriage-and-health literature is that couples should first work to repair a troubled relationship and learn to fight without hostility and derision. But if staying married means living amid constant acrimony, from the point of view of your health, "you're better off out of it," she says.

Last year, The Journal of Health and Social Behavior published a study tracking the marital history and health of nearly 9,000 men and women in their 50s and 60s. The study, which grew out of work by researchers at the University of Chicago, found that when the married people became single again — either by divorce or because of the death of a spouse — they suffered a decline in physical health from which they never fully recovered. These men and women had 20 percent more chronic health issues, like heart disease and diabetes, than those who were still married to their first husband or wife by middle age. The divorced and widowed also had aged less gracefully, reporting more problems going up and down stairs or walking longer distances.

Perhaps the most striking finding concerned single people who had never married. For more than 100 years, scientists have speculated that single people, because they generally have fewer resources, lower income and perhaps less logistical and emotional support, have poorer health than the married. But in the Chicago study, people who had divorced or been widowed had worse health problems than men and women who had been single their entire lives. In formerly married individuals, it was as if the marriage advantage had never existed.

Does marrying again benefit those who divorce, in terms of health? In the Chicago study, remarriage helped only a little. It seemed to heal emotional wounds: the remarried had about the same risk for depression as the continuously married. But a second marriage didn't seem to be enough to repair the physical damage associated with marital loss. Compared with the continuously married, people in second marriages still had 12 percent more chronic health problems and 19 percent more mobility problems. "I don't think anyone would encourage people to stay in a marriage that is really making them miserable," says Linda J. Waite, a University of Chicago sociologist and an author of the study. "But try harder to make it better." Even if marital problems seem small, Waite says, the data suggest it's wise to intervene early and try to resolve them. "If you learn to how to manage disagreement early," she says, "then you can avoid the decline in marital happiness that follows from the drip, drip of negative interactions."

Other researchers have also studied how the "drip, drip" of negativity can erode not only a marriage itself but also a couple's physical health. A number of epidemiological studies suggest that unhappily married couples are at higher risk for heart attacks and cardiovascular disease than happily married couples. In 2000, The Journal of the American Medical Association published a three-year Swedish study of 300 women who had been hospitalized with severe chest pains or a heart attack; the study found that those who reported the highest levels of marital stress were nearly three times as likely to suffer another heart attack or require a bypass or other procedure. It is notable that these increased risks weren't associated with other forms of stress. For instance, women who were stressed-out at work weren't at any higher risk for a second episode of heart problems than women who were happy in their jobs.

Of course, all couples — happy or unhappy — are bound to experience some form of marital conflict. Surely this does not mean everyone is doomed to ill health; some conflicts are better than others. The University of Utah psychology professor Timothy W. Smith has addressed this question, studying how what he calls the "emotional tone" of conflict affects heart risk. In one study, he recruited 150 couples, most of whom were in their 60s and married for an average of 36 years. All were in general good health with no signs of heart disease. Smith collected video recordings of the couples discussing stressful topics like money management or housework.

The arguments were then "coded" to indicate the number of warm, hostile and controlling statements and words that were used in the course of the dispute. In addition, the couples were put in heart-scanning machines to measure coronary calcium levels, which are a useful indicator of heart-disease risk. Smith then compared each person's conflict style with their coronary calcium score.

Smith's results suggest that there are important differences between men and women when it comes to health and the style of conflict that can jeopardize it. The women in his study who were at highest risk for signs of heart disease were those whose marital battles lacked any signs of warmth, not even a stray term of endearment during a hostile discussion ("*Honey*, you're driving me crazy!") or a minor pat on the back or squeeze of the hand, all of which can signal affection in the midst of anger. "Most of the literature assumes that it's how bad the arguments get that drives the effect, but it's actually the lack of affection that does it," Smith told me. "It wasn't how much nasty talk there was. It was the lack of warmth that predicted risk."

For men, on the other hand, hostile and negative marital battles seemed to have no effect on heart risk. Men were at risk for a higher coronary calcium score, however, when their marital spats turned into battles for *control*. It didn't matter whether it was the husband or wife who was trying to gain control of the matter; it was merely any appearance of controlling language that put men on the path of heart disease.

In both cases, the emotional tone of a marital fight turned out to be just as predictive of poor heart health as whether the individual smoked or had high cholesterol. It is worth noting that the couples in Smith's study were all relatively happy. These were husbands and wives who loved each other. Yet many of them had developed styles of conflict that took a physical toll on each other. The solution, Smith noted, isn't to stop fighting. It's to fight more thoughtfully. "Difficulties in marriage seem to be nearly universal," he said. "Just try not to let fights be any nastier than they need to be."

Researchers have also started to examine the salutary health effects of social relationships, including those of a good marriage. In one recent study, James A. Coan, an assistant professor of psychology and a neuroscientist at the University of Virginia, recruited 16 women who scored relatively high on a questionnaire assessing marital happiness. He placed each woman in three different situations while monitoring her brain with an f.M.R.I. machine, which offers a way to observe the brain's response to almost any kind of emotional stimulation. In one situation, to simulate stress, he subjected the woman to a mild electric shock. In a second, the shock was administered, but the woman held the hand of a stranger; in a third, the hand of her husband.

Both instances of hand-holding reduced the neural activity in areas of the woman's brain associated with stress. But when the woman was holding her husband's hand, the effect was even greater, and it was particularly pronounced in women who had the highest marital-happiness scores. Holding a husband's hand during the electric shock resulted in a calming of the brain regions associated with pain similar to the effect brought about by use of a pain-relieving drug.

Coan says the study simulates how a supportive marriage and partnership gives the brain the opportunity to outsource some of its most difficult neural work. "When someone holds your hand in a study or just shows that they are there for you by giving you a back rub, when you're in their presence, that becomes a cue that you don't have to regulate your negative emotion," he told me. "The other person is essentially regulating your negative emotion but without your prefrontal cortex. It's much less wear and tear on us if we have someone there to help regulate us."

With so much evidence establishing a link between marital stress and health, a new generation of research is set to explore the ways in which couples can mitigate the damaging effects of relationship stress. The Glasers are now conducting studies testing whether regular supplements of fish oil, rich in omega-3 fatty acids, can mitigate some of the physical symptoms of stress on the immune system.

The couple are also embarking on a new study looking at the interplay between nutrition and marital stress. Earlier research at Ohio State showed that when study subjects were given intravenous fat injections during times of stress, it took longer for triglycerides, fats that are associated with heart disease, to leave the bloodstream. But Kiecolt-Glaser is more interested in the real-world equivalent of the study: What happens to the body's ability to cope with fats when couples fight at dinnertime? To find out, she's planning to feed married couples two types of meals — one relatively healthful meal and one high-fat meal equivalent to fast food. During the meal the couples will be asked to discuss topics of high stress, and a blood analysis will offer a glimpse of the effect that mealtime conflict has on the body's ability to metabolize fats. "It's an ideal way," Kiecolt-Glaser says, "to look at what happens to couples in the real world, where so many family conflicts happen over a meal."

For the Glasers, their nearly 30 years of professional collaboration have not only given them new insights into the role of stress and health but have also helped them in their own marriage. Like every married couple, they have their disagreements, Glaser told me. But years of watching married couples interact and measuring the subsequent physical toll that conflict takes on their bodies has taught the Glasers the importance of taking time off together and making sure their disagreements don't degenerate into personal attacks. "Don't fight dirty," he advised. "You never go far enough down the road where you hurt each other. We know enough to avoid those kinds of arguments."

Kiecolt-Glaser added that the couple's research shows that some level of relationship stress is inevitable in even the happiest marriages. The important thing, she said, is to use those moments of stress as an opportunity to repair the relationship rather than to damage it. "It can be so uncomfortable, even in the best marriages, to have an ongoing disagreement," she said. "It's the pit-in-your-stomach kind of thing. But when your marital relationship is the key relationship in your life, a disagreement is really a signal to try to fix something."

Tara Parker-Pope is the Well columnist for The New York Times and the author of "For Better: The Science of a Good Marriage."

Appendix G:
Glamour Magazine Article

Shocking Body-Image News: 97% of Women Will Be Cruel to Their Bodies Today

by Shaun Dreisbach

Read these words: "You are a fat, worthless pig." "You're too thin. No man is ever going to want you." "Ugly. Big. Gross." Horrifying comments on some awful website? The rant of an abusive, controlling boyfriend? No; shockingly, these are the actual words young women are saying to themselves on any typical day. For some, such thoughts are fleeting, but for others, this dialogue plays on a constant, punishing loop, according to a new exclusive *Glamour* survey of more than 300 women of all sizes. Our research found that, on average, women have 13 negative body thoughts daily—nearly one for every waking hour. And a disturbing number of women confess to having 35, 50 or even 100 hateful thoughts about their own shapes each day.

Our experiment went like this: We challenged young women across the country to note every negative or anxious thought they had about their bodies over the course of one full day. The results shocked us: A whopping *97 percent* admitted to having at least one "I hate my body" moment.

"That is *a lot*, yet I'm not totally surprised," says Ann Kearney-Cooke, Ph.D., a Cincinnati psychologist who specializes in body image and helped *Glamour* design the survey. "It's become such an accepted norm to put yourself down that if someone says she likes her body, she's the odd woman out. I was in a group discussion recently, and when one woman said, 'I actually feel OK about the way I look,' another woman scrunched up her face and said, 'I have never in my whole life heard anyone say that—and I'm not sure I even believe you.' That's how pervasive this negative body talk is. It's actually more acceptable to insult your body than to praise it."

And we seem to be well aware of how hard we are on ourselves. Nearly 63 percent of Glamour's survey respondents said they had roughly the same number of negative thoughts as they expected. But few realized how venomous those thoughts were until they were down on paper. So how has this become OK?

Our unattainable cultural beauty ideals, our celebrity worship—those all play a part, says Kearney-Cooke. But another big reason is that we've actually *trained* ourselves to be this way. "Neuroscience has shown that whatever you focus on shapes your brain. If you're constantly thinking negative thoughts about your body, that neural pathway becomes stronger—and those thoughts become habitual," she explains. "Imagine a concert pianist. Her brain would have stronger neural pathways that support musicality and dexterity than someone who hadn't spent her life practicing."

Our "training" begins early. In a University of Central Florida study of three- to six-year-old girls, nearly half were already worried about being fat—and roughly a third said they wanted to change something about their body. "There are only so many times you can be hit with the message that your body isn't 'right'— whether you see it on TV, hear it from your mom or just feel it in the ether—before you internalize it and start beating yourself up for not being as perfect as you 'should' be," says Nichole Wood—Barcalow, Ph.D., a psychologist at the Laureate Eating Disorders Program in Tulsa, Oklahoma. As Maureen Dorsett, 28, of Washington, D.C., who counted 11 negative thoughts the day she did our experiment, puts it: "I always saw my negative thoughts as a way of improving myself—of calling attention to what I need to work on. If a guy said to me, 'Wow, your belly looks flabby today,' that would be really offensive.

Somehow, these thoughts never seemed as degrading coming from my own mind. Maybe I had just gotten so used to having them."

To make matters worse, negative talk has become part of the way women bond. "Friends getting together and tearing themselves down is such a common thing that it's hard to avoid," says Kearney-Cooke. The chatter happens on Facebook and among coworkers, and is broadcast with surprising viciousness on shows like *Real Housewives* and *Bridalplasty* (on which one perfectly cute contestant declared, "I want this butt face fixed!"). And all that public bashing makes the internal insult-athon seem normal. As one woman told us, "When others make comments about their bodies, it makes me think about *mine* more."

Hmm. If our brains are virtually wired this way—and outside cultural forces aren't helping—how can we stop the self-hate? We were determined to find out.

Why Your Body May Not Be the Problem

When *Glamour* analyzed the data to look for a cause of these ruthless thoughts, a fascinating trend emerged: Respondents who were unsatisfied with their career or relationship tended to report more negative body thoughts than women who were content in those areas. What's more, feeling uncomfortable emotions of any sort—stress, loneliness, even boredom—made many women start berating their looks. "If we're having a bad day, we often take those negative emotions out on our body, rather than directing them at what's really troubling us, like our boss or boyfriend," says Wood-Barcalow. In fact—and this part's important—whether you're unhappy in general is a much larger factor in how you feel about your body than what your body actually *looks*like. In our survey, thin and average-weight women were just as likely to insult themselves as overweight ones. As Wood-Barcalow recites to her patients: "It's all about your body—and absolutely nothing about your body."

Consider: "Let's say you're in a meeting and you suddenly think, Ew, my arms are huge," says Kearney-Cooke. "Well, you've had those same arms all day. Why are you suddenly feeling bad about them now? Maybe it's because you don't think your professional ideas are being valued or you're not fulfilled in your job. Instead of focusing on the real issue, all you can think of is hating your arms. And it becomes a vicious cycle: All the push-ups in the world won't make you feel better, because your arms weren't the problem to begin with."

Silencing Your Inner "Mean Girl"

So how can you muzzle that insulting internal voice and get on with your life? "I'm way too hard on myself, but I don't know how to lessen my negative thoughts," admits Rebecca Illson, 25, of Birmingham, Michigan, who counted 50 of them over the course of the day. And that age-old advice to "love your body" is—let's be honest—trite and unhelpful. "It's not about achieving a 'perfect' body image. That's not realistic," says Wood-Barcalow. "Even the most confident women have doubts. But they've learned to combat those thoughts rather than allow them to take over."

It's worth it for not just the mental peace but your *physical* health as well. Research at the University of British Columbia, Vancouver, suggests that women who obsess over their body and diet have chronically elevated levels of the stress hormone cortisol (even when their life is *not* otherwise stressed)—and, as a result, may suffer from elevated blood pressure, lower bone density, higher amounts of unhealthy belly fat and even menstrual problems. "And this was among women in their twenties!" exclaims lead researcher Jennifer Bedford, Ph.D. "If you continue on this path, it could have a real impact on heart, bone and reproductive health 10 or 20 years down the road."

Hope for Real Change

Not convinced *you* can stop the snark? Wood-Barcalow thinks you can. She recently conducted one of the few studies of young women with good body image—and was surprised to discover that 80 percent of them had struggled with negative body thoughts earlier in their life. "The fact that they were able to boost themselves up is proof that it's possible for *all* women to adopt a better outlook on their body." Here, seven ways to do just that:

1. Rewire your brain. If you know that constantly thinking negatively about your body teaches your brain to focus on the bad stuff, why not flip the script? "It's absolutely possible to create neural pathways that favor affirming thoughts," says Kearney-Cooke. She suggests keeping a pen handy to note things you do that make you feel *good* about your body. "One of my patients is doing this, and she came in so excited to tell me, 'Look at my list now: It's so big!' Doing this puts positive stuff front-of-mind and starts becoming instinctive."

2. Ask yourself: Is this *really* about my body? Or am I trying to distract myself from being upset with someone or something else? This is another exercise Kearney-Cooke does with women. "I had a patient who came in and lamented, 'My body is disgusting today!' After she stopped to think about it for a minute, she realized it wasn't about her body at all. She admitted she got drunk the night before and was embarrassed about it. That's the issue she needs to address—drinking too much—not the size of her butt."

3. Exercise! Survey respondents who worked out regularly tended to report fewer harsh thoughts than those who didn't. And it's not just that being physically active improves your shape and health; it actually boosts your mind-set, too. One new study found that women felt better about themselves after exercising even when their bodies didn't change, suggesting that the feeling of "That was challenging, and I did it!" played a bigger role than weight loss in boosting body image. "Hitting the gym or horseback riding makes me feel like a fitness rock star. It's the biggest confidence booster for me," says Margo Short, 22, of Dallas, who counted four negative thoughts—about two-thirds *fewer* than the average respondent. (For a workout you can do at home, <u>click here</u>.)

4. Say "stop!"—literally, that word—when your mind goes all negative. "Just imagine a giant screaming stop sign," says Kearney-Cooke. Emily Catalano, 22, of Boston, who logged just three bad body thoughts, does this: "It's funny, but it really does shut up that negative voice and clears my head."

5. Remind yourself that obsessing about what you eat or look like doesn't make you *look* any better. Bedford's study found that young women who obsess over their diet don't actually weigh less than those who generally eat what they want. "Some women look at a brownie and think: Ooh, that looks good, but brownies are 'bad'. I wonder how many calories are in that? Maybe I could just have a teeny bite, and on and on. A woman with a healthier relationship with food would either eat the brownie, or not, and be done," explains Bedford. At the end of the day, both get the same number of calories. The message: Fretting over every bite gets you nowhere. Eating mindfully—enjoying food and putting your fork down before you get too full—feels better *and* works better.

6. Appreciate your body for what it does, rather than how it looks. In our survey, 55 percent of women had abusive thoughts about their overall weight or size; 43 percent said they targeted specific areas (the most berated: belly and thighs). "Next time you're, say, cursing your wobbly arms, pause and think of their purpose—is it to make you feel bad? Or to let you hug your friends and enjoy life?" says Wood-Barcalow. It may seem a bit "Kumbaya," but this mental tweak helped many respondents think less negatively. Jenni Schaefer, 34, of Austin, Texas, who reported only two bad body thoughts on the day in question, points to her ability to "be grateful that I can walk and that my body is healthy."

7. Finally, play up your strengths. "Comparing yourself with others doesn't help anything," reminds Kearney-Cooke. "Focus on making the most of what you've got. Hold your head a little higher and walk a little taller: That attitude is absolutely magnetic." Hear that? You're *magnetic*. And don't forget to tell yourself so, either. We all could use a few more compliments!

The Real (Really Harsh) Things Women Think About Their Bodies

If a man talked this way to a woman, it would be considered relationship abuse. So why do we spew such venom at ourselves? Brace yourself and listen to the real thoughts of women *Glamour* surveyed.

"Fat-ass. Lazy bitch. I hate my thighs. I hate my stomach. I hate my arms."

"Don't eat that. You could probably use an eating disorder."

"Your stomach is fat. That is why you are alone."

"Oh my God, look at her waist and legs! We're the same height. She looks like a model. I look like a lumpy sock."

"You're obese. All the pretty girls are size 2."

"I can't imagine anyone wanting to have sex with this."

"Scrawny and messed up."

"You're bigger than her. Fatty."

"Big nose, disgusting skin, bags under eyes, ugly feet, small breasts."

"Please don't let my size 00 coworker notice this huge gut I've been cultivating."

"You look like an Oompa-Loompa."

"Huge legs, fat stomach, not pretty enough to attract anyone, ugly in comparison to others."

"I look disgusting with my cottage cheese legs and stretch-mark hips. Nasty. No one would want to touch me."

"I'm ugly. Too skinny. Look sick."

EARTH TO WOMEN: Stop this madness! We deserve better than this. If you wouldn't say it to a friend, don't say it to yourself.

Secrets of the 3% of Women Who Love Their Bodies

That's the minuscule proportion of the women we surveyed who said they had no negative body thoughts the day they did our experiment. So what's in their water?

"I struggled with my body image when I was younger. I'm of Bangladeshi descent, and when I was growing up, other girls were always thinner, blonder and more perfect and popular. I finally had this turning point where I actually decided to just give up. It sounds crazy, but I remember thinking I was so tired of trying to fit in and beating myself up and getting nowhere. I thought life couldn't possibly get worse if I just gave up and decided to be myself. And you know what? I realized that there really was no change in my quality of life whether I was a little heavier or at the 'perfect' weight. I was still happy and successful and boys liked me and my friends loved me. Now I know what is healthy for me."
—*Tasneem Alam, 25, New York City*

"I want people around me who are positive. I had a boss once who actually used to make comments about my being small (I'm 5'1" and 100 pounds), saying, 'Why are you wearing that? It makes you look even more like a toothpick.' It took my coworkers' assuring me that it wasn't about me, but about how my boss felt about herself. Now, I'd still love to be taller and curvier. But you know what? Only so many women in the world can be Victoria's Secret models. I have to appreciate myself the way I am."
—*Karen Hudson, 31, Moore, Okla.*

"I remind myself of what I have control over. For example, you can't control the fact that things naturally get a little softer as you age, but you can feed your body healthy food and stay active. You can't make your curly hair straight no matter how many irons you take to it, but you *can* have your stylist show you how to rock your natural texture. Taking ownership of your choices gives you power. I'm never going to look in the mirror and see a blond surfer girl, but neither is Christina Hendricks, Zooey Deschanel or Janelle Monae. Those are all stunning women who stand out because they aren't trying to alter their true nature."
—*Marie-Gael Gray, 30, Athens, Ohio*

Bibliography

Castillo, Stephanie. "You'll Have a Better Orgasm With Foreplay, Finds The Least Surprising Study Ever." *Prevention.com* March 2014. http://www.prevention.com/sex/sex-relationships/youll-have-better-orgasm-foreplay-finds-least-surprising-study-ever.

Dreisbach, Shaun. "Shocking Body-Image News: 97% of Women Will Be Cruel to Their Bodies Today." *Glamour.com* February 2011. http://www.glamour.com/health-fitness/2011/02/shocking-body-image-news-97-percent-of-women-will-be-cruel-to-their-bodies-today/1.

Pitt, Brad, Anthony Hopkins, and Claire Forlani. *Meet Joe Black*. Directed by Martin Brest. Hollywood, CA: Universal Studios, 1998.

271

Smith, Davey G., S. Frankel, and J. Yarnel. "Sex and death: are they related? Findings from the Caerphilly Cohort Study." *British Medical Journal* 1997 Dec 20-27; 315(7123):1641-4, accessed June 2013, http://www.ncbi.nlm.nih.gov/pubmed/9448525.

Thank You

Thank you for purchasing this book and transforming your life and relationship.

Please check out the link below to access a free video series we've made to assist and deepen your desire to be and feel more love in your life; a perfect primer to utilizing this book as the short videos will highlight the most powerful tools and issues to ensure you create the love life of your dreams!

InLoveForever.tv

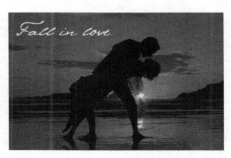

If you are interested in taking the fast path toward being *In Love Forever* and are ready and desiring to commit time, energy, and resources into transforming your life – whether that's to improve your relationship or to get into a one – you are invited to see if you qualify for a **50 minute complimentary Revitalize Your Love & Passion Session** ($350 value) offered by Cary Valentine and the exceptional *In Love Forever* coaching team.

In this session, we will:

1) Create a clear vision of the kind of relationship you want.

2) Assist you in determining the essential relationship skills you desire to improve.

3) Discover the #1 factor slowing you down or stopping you from having the relationship of your dreams.

4) Identify the actions that will quickly move you forward into the relationship vision you created.

5) Complete the session with excitement knowing what to do next to create and experience the relationship of your dreams.

Contact us at: WeCare@InLoveForever.com

Mention "Qualify for a Revitalize Your Love & Passion Session" in the subject line.